Keto Diet After 50

The Complete Guide to Ketogenic Diet for Men and Women Over 50...Includes Quick and Easy Recipes for Losing Weight and Many Meal Plans

Jacob Richie

Table of Contents

Chapter 5: Easy Keto Breakfast Recipes 64

Chapter 6: Easy Keto Lunch Recipes 107

Chapter 9: Easy Keto Dessert Recipes 229

Introduction

Congratulations on buying *Keto Diet After 50*. Thanks a lot for doing so.

There are various types of diet plans that can be found today for losing weight. But, there are only a few diet plans that are effective even after the age of 50. The ketogenic diet falls under this group. This diet plan is based on low carb consumption. If you are above the age of 50 and willing to start with a proper diet plan, this book has all the information you need. The keto diet is very effective in losing weight, besides keeping you healthy and fit. When you get the opportunity to start with a proper diet plan that perfectly suits your age group, building your long-desired body will become easier, and so will its maintenance. If you are not familiar with a low carb diet, starting with the keto diet might sound a bit tough. However, with time as you get the desired results, it will become easier for you.

The keto diet meal plans are often treated as being controversial. The primary reason behind this is most people think the high-fat content of the meals can increase the body's cholesterol level. However, according to some recent studies, following a diet low on carbs has its own benefits. The recipes you will come across in this book can help start with the keto diet very easily.

You can find lots of books based on this subject in today's market. Thank you again for selecting this one! Every effort was given to make sure this book is filled with as much beneficial information as possible. So, please enjoy it!

Chapter 1: How to Begin With a Keto Diet After 50

The ketogenic diet is a long-known diet plan that is very effective in losing extra weight. It is low in carbs and is high in fat consumption. It has been found that the keto diet is can in improving the quality of your health besides shedding extra weight. It can impart several other types of benefits on the body against epilepsy, diabetes, cancer, and Alzheimer's disease. Several studies found that the keto diet is more popular among women as it can show positive results in dealing with the various symptoms of menopause. Some of the most common menopause symptoms are irritability, fatigue, and sudden increase in body weight. Various researches claim that the keto diet can very easily deal with all these symptoms. But is it really so? Are you thinking of starting with the diet but not sure where to start from? This section has got all that you need.

Basics About the Keto Diet

The keto diet or ketogenic diet is a low-carb diet. It has several similarities with the low-carb and Atkins diet. The main aim of this diet is to reduce your intake of carbohydrates drastically. You will need to replace the same with healthy fats. As you reduce the consumption of carbohydrates drastically, the body will enter a metabolic state. This state is known as ketosis. When ketosis occurs, your body will become more efficient in burning out all the fat to provide energy to the body for carrying out various basic functions. It will also turn the body fats into ketones in your liver that helps supply the required energy to the brain. The keto diet also reduces the levels of insulin and blood sugar drastically. This, in addition to the increased number of ketones, comes with several other health benefits.

Ketogenic Diet for Losing Weight

The keto diet is a very effective and easy way of losing extra pounds from your body. It also helps to cut off the risk factors of various diseases. It has been found that this diet is even more effective than various other low-fat diets. Additionally, the keto diet is so filling in nature that you will be able to shed all the extra weight without counting on calories or keeping track of food consumption. In a study, it has been stated that people who follow the keto diet can lose about two times more weight in comparison to those people who are on a calorie-restricted and low-fat diet. The HDL cholesterol level, along with the levels of triglyceride, also gets improved.

Ketogenic Diet for Prediabetes and Diabetes

Diabetes is most often characterized by various metabolic state changes, impaired functioning of insulin, and high blood sugar levels. The keto diet can reduce excess fat, which can be linked to metabolic syndrome, type 2 diabetes, and prediabetes. According to the latest study, this diet plan can improve sensitivity to insulin by almost 75%. So, it can be said that this diet can easily help in dealing with diabetes, along with its various characteristics.

Several Other Health Benefits Related to the Keto Diet

There are various other benefits of the keto diet besides weight loss and dealing with diabetes.

- **Cancer:** This diet plan is now being adapted to treat various cancer types and slow tumor growth.

- **Alzheimer's disease:** According to recent studies, the keto diet can help in dealing with Alzheimer's disease and slow its progression speed.

- **Polycystic ovary syndrome:** The keto diet effectively reduces insulin levels, which can play an important role in reducing polycystic ovary syndrome.

- **Increase in the level of HDL cholesterol:** HDL cholesterol is known as good cholesterol. The keto diet can increase HDL levels by lowering the intake of carbohydrates and consuming more fats. This will help to lower the risks of various heart-related diseases or even heart attacks.

- **Better sleep:** It has been found that even a small quantity of glucose in the diet is very effective in disturbing the blood sugar levels in the body. It will ultimately lead to poor or bad sleep. As you grow with age, the quality of sleep is most likely to degrade. When you start following the keto diet, it can help keep blood sugar levels under proper control. Additionally, it can also help balance the levels of other types of hormones like cortisol and melatonin.

-

How Can You Easily Start the Diet?

Adapting the keto diet is not at all tough. However, you will need to take care of certain things for the best possible results.

- **Having a clear idea of what foods to consume and what to avoid:** It is very important to understand what food items you can consume and whatnot. You will need to concentrate on limiting the intake of carbs with more focus on healthy fats.

- **Examine your connection with healthy fats:** For starting with a diet high in fats, you will need to start with very small adjustments. It might turn out to be uncomfortable at the beginning. But, making small changes every day can help in easing the process for you.

- **Plan a starting date:** A very important thing that you will need to ensure is to sort out your entire diet schedule. Start by fixing a date and start from that day only. In case you have any parties or other plans with your friends, try to share your target with them. It will help you to get all the support you need for starting with the diet plan.

- **Limiting the daily carbohydrate intake to 20 grams:** As you start to push your body towards ketosis, it is very important for you that you start consuming lots of healthy fats. As the ketogenic diet's primary motive is to lower the intake of carbohydrates, make sure that your daily intake of carbs does not go beyond 20 grams. It is a very important step. What you can do is that you can add more fat along with proteins for filling up that space. Maintaining the ratio of carbs to fat is very important for supplying the body with the required amount of ketones.

Chapter 2: Why Is It Hard to Lose Weight After 50 and Effects of Aging on Nutritional Needs

All those diets that worked out so well during your 20s, 30s, or 40s do not seem to work like before after crossing the mark of 50. Why so? Are you not hitting your treadmill hard or consuming too many carbs? Losing weight after the age of 50 and beyond is a completely different game. You might think that it is very hard or impossible to shed those extra pounds after 50. But, you still have the opportunity to eliminate those extra pounds. All you need to do is determine all those hurdles that are standing in front of you.

You Are Experiencing Muscle Loss Due to Age

The total amount of lean muscle that you have naturally will start to decline by 4 to 7 percent every decade after crossing the mark of 30. This process is known as sarcopenia. You might also start losing muscles if you are not that active because of various health conditions related to age, such as arthritis. Getting a surgery or injury after 30 can also lead to the same. All of these instances might not lead to any significant kind of decline. However, cumulatively, they all do. Why does muscle loss matter? The main logic behind this is that the lean muscles tend to use up more calories than fat. So, if you are not training your strength daily with weights for building and maintaining muscle, there will be fewer needs of calories every day. It can lead to weight gain if you keep consuming the same number of calories exactly like when you were younger.

Majority of the people have the tendency not to adjust their calorie consumption as they age. They will just keep on eating the same. As they possess lean muscle mass for burning all those calories and less percentage of activity, the result is weight gain.

Normal Changes in Hormone Levels

Every human being undergoes several changes in their levels of hormones as a normal part of their aging. It can easily explain why mid-age is the pick time of putting on extra pounds. For women, the onset of menopause, which typically occurs between the age of forty-five and fifty-five, results in a drastic drop in estrogen levels. This tends to encourage the accumulation of extra pounds near the belly very easily. This kind of shift in the storage of fats can make the gain of weight even more noticeable. It can also make a sudden rise in the overall risk of high blood pressure, heart disease, diabetes, and high cholesterol. Also, fluctuations in estrogen levels during perimenopause, the years before menopause, can result in mood swings. This kind of sudden mood swings might make it tougher to just stick to an exercise plan along with a healthy diet.

For men, there is a sudden change in the levels of testosterone with age. The testosterone level tends to decline gradually around the age of 40 by two to three percent every year. Besides other things, testosterone is responsible for regulating fat distribution along with muscle mass and strength. In simple terms, reduction in testosterone levels can result in making the body less effective in burning calories.

With age, the growth hormone which is produced by the pituitary gland also reduces in percentage. One of the primary functions of the growth hormone is to maintain and build muscle mass. So, when the level of growth hormone decreases, it gets tougher for the body to build and maintain the mass of muscles.

The Rate of Metabolism Becomes Slow

When there is a decrease in muscle mass, the body's metabolic rate tends to slow down. Metabolism is a very complex process that helps in the conversion of calories into useful energy. Having less muscle and more fat will reduce the calorie-burning process. Also, many people tend to get less active with growing age. It can also slow down the metabolism. Age is not the primary thing that can determine the metabolic rate. The sex and size of the body also play important roles. Certain types of health conditions, like hypothyroidism, can also affect the rate of metabolism.

More Stress and Less Activity

As you reach the age of fifty, your work schedule or career is most likely to be in full swing. This can lead to certain challenges in weight loss. You will be moving less, commute to your work by seating for an hour and work at the desk for seven or more hours. You will already have so much served on the plate that you will find it difficult to take out some time for exercise or a short walk during the day. With more work pressure, you will get more stress as well. It can result in a sudden boost in ghrelin levels, the hormone that can make you hungrier. You will end up consuming more calories. Ultimately this will lead to weight increase.

Not Enough Sleep

Not getting enough sleep and sleep disturbances are very common as you cross the mark of 50. For women, menopause can lead to sleep disruptions because of hot flashes or even arthritis. When you do not get enough sleep, it readily affects the overall production of the growth hormone. Growth hormone is essential for muscle and bone mass.

Relation Between Aging and Nutritional Needs

While talking about aging, it can be related to several types of body changes, for instance, muscle loss, thinner skin, less stomach acid, and many others.

Most of these can lead to nutrient deficiency, while others might directly affect the quality of life and the senses. For instance, it has been found that approximately 27% of elderly people tend to suffer from atrophic gastritis. It is a condition that leads to the chronic nature of inflammation along with cellular damage. All of these are responsible for the production of stomach acid. As the level of acid in our stomach gets low, it can readily affect the absorption of nutrients like vitamin B12, iron, calcium, and magnesium.

Malnutrition can be treated as both a consequence and a cause of ill health. It might be of several types, such as overnutrition, undernutrition, or even specific nutrition deficiencies. Malnutrition in aging people, is most of the time, underdiagnosed. Malnutrition in people who have crossed the 50 mark can result in various health problems and a weaker immune system. When you tend to have a weak immune system, there is most likely to be an increase in the risk of infections, muscle weakness, and poor healing of wounds.

Including More Fiber in Daily Diet

Constipation is among the most common problems that can be found in elderly people. Constipation is more common among all those people who are above the age of 50. According to some studies, women tend to suffer more from constipation as compared to men. The development of constipation, along with growing age, comes along with a definite reason. As with growing age, you are most likely to have lesser movements. You might also need to consume various types of medications. In such cases, constipation might develop as a definite side effect. But, how to get rid of this? The solution is simple. You will need to consume more fiber. Fiber can very easily pass through the gut even in its undigested form. So, it can help in the proper passing of stool with even movements of the bowel. Also, as you start consuming more fiber, it can help in the prevention of diverticular disease. It is a serious condition in which various small structures develop along the colon wall.

Need for More Nutrients and Fewer Calories

The daily amount of calories needed by a person relies on several factors like weight, activity level, muscle mass, height, and various others. Elderly adults and people above the age of 50 require fewer calories. The primary reason behind this is less amount of exercise and lesser movements. When you continue consuming the same number of calories per day, just like the days when you were younger, it will result in fat gain. The fat gain can be seen mainly near the belly area. Although the need for calories is much less, there is a high need for various other types of nutrients. That is why people above the age of 50 need to consume several types of whole food items such as lean meat, fish, and veggies. Whole food can help in dealing with a deficiency of nutrients without any effect on the waistline. Some examples of essential nutrients are vitamin B12, vitamin D, calcium, protein, and others.

Increased Need for Vitamin B12

Vitamin B12 belongs to the group of essential nutrients that are required with growing age. The most important function carried out by this vitamin is the production of red blood cells. Not only that, but vitamin B12 is also responsible for proper brain functioning. According to some recent studies, about 25-30% of people who have crossed the 50 mark are most likely to have reduced ability to absorb vitamin B12 from the diet they follow. So, with passing time, it can eventually lead to vitamin B12 deficiency. Vitamin B12 comes along with all those proteins that we consume daily. Before the body can use up this vitamin, the stomach acids help separate the same from the proteins. With growing age, the production of acid in the stomach is most likely to decrease. So, this might result in lesser absorption of this important vitamin from our daily diet.

Importance of Calcium and Vitamin D

We all know that vitamin D, along with calcium, is essential for maintaining the bones' proper health. Calcium is responsible for building up and maintenance of healthy bones. On the other hand, vitamin D helps in the absorption of calcium by the body. However, elderly people can absorb less amount of calcium from their daily diet. It has been found that the gut tends to absorb less calcium with growing age.

But, the primary reason behind the decrease in calcium absorption is vitamin D deficiency. Vitamin D can be produced by the human body from the available cholesterol in the skin when exposed to the sunlight. As we grow old, our skin also becomes thinner. So, the ability of the skin to produce vitamin D also gets reduced.

So, because of vitamin D and calcium deficiency, our bone health will also decrease. Thus, the risk of fractures and injuries will tend to increase. Green leafy vegetables, along with dairy products, are great sources of calcium. Vitamin D is available in several types of fish like salmon, herring, and others.

There are several other types of nutrients that you will need with growing age. Some of them are:

- **Magnesium:** This nutrient aids in the process of digestion as it tends to get disrupted with age. It is very important besides vitamin and calcium.

- **Potassium:** As you increase the consumption of potassium, the risks of osteoporosis, kidney stones, heart diseases, and high blood pressure will also get reduced.

- **Iron:** Deficiency of iron can lead to anemia, which is very common in elderly people. It is a condition where oxygen is deficient in the blood.

- **Omega-3 fatty acid:** It is very important for heart health. It can also help in lowering high blood pressure.

With growing age, maintaining a proper proportion of nutrients is very important. The diet that you will choose will determine the kind of life that you will have.

Chapter 3: Keto Diet Food List

The ketogenic diet is all about restricting the consumption of carbohydrates. Typically, carbs are regarded as the preferred energy source of the body. However, when you are on a strict keto diet, the energy intake from carbs will be even less than five percent. That is what triggers the process of ketosis in the body. Even when you have a clear idea that you will need to concentrate on eating high-fat low-carb food items, it might still turn out to be a bit confusing as to which food items you can eat. In this chapter, you will find most of the food items you can consume while on a ketogenic diet.

Seafood and Fish

Fish is a great source of selenium, B vitamins, and potassium. Additionally, it is rich in proteins and is free from carbs as well. Sardines, salmons, albacore tuna, mackerel, and other fatty fish types come with a great percentage of omega-3 fatty acids. If you want to lower your blood sugar levels, omega-3 fatty acids can help you a lot. It can also increase the sensitivity to insulin. Frequent fish consumption can be linked with a decreased risk of various types of chronic diseases and great mental health.

Low-Carb Vegetables

Non-starchy vegetables are low in carbs as well as calories. They are rich in various types of nutrients, like vitamin C and essential minerals. Low-carb veggies are rich in antioxidants that can help in protecting against the free radicals that damage cells. You can aim to consume non-starchy veggies with about eight grams of net carbs for each cup. Some great options for low-carb veggies are cauliflower, broccoli, bell peppers, green beans, spinach, and zucchini. You can very easily substitute high-carb foods with vegetables. For instance, cauliflower can be used in place of rice or mashed potatoes, or you can also substitute noodles with zoodles made from zucchini and many others.

Cheese

Cheese falls under the group of food items that are tasty and rich in nutrients as well. There are various cheese types that can be found in the market. Fortunately, cheeses of all types are high in fat and are low in carbs. So, you can consider cheese as a perfect food item that can be included in your ketogenic diet plan. Consuming one ounce of cheese can provide your body with seven grams of protein, one gram of carbs, and fifteen percent RDI for calcium. Majority of the people think of cheese as being unhealthy as it is rich in saturated fat. However, cheese consumption has still not shown any sign in increasing the overall risk of heart diseases. Additionally, cheese also comes with linoleic acid, which is most often related to fat loss. Cheese is a great food item that can help in muscle mass retention, which generally reduces with growing age.

Avocado

Avocado can be included in your ketogenic diet plan as a heart-healthy fat. It is rich in potassium and fat. Consuming half an avocado will provide you with only nine grams of carbs, out of which seven grams are fiber. Shifting to plant fats from animal fats can help in readily improving the levels of triglyceride and cholesterol.

Eggs

Eggs are a great source of minerals, proteins, B vitamins, and antioxidants. Consuming two eggs every day will provide you with zero carbs and twelve grams of protein. Eggs can trigger hormones that can help to increase the feeling of fullness. It can also help in stabilizing the levels of blood sugar. Eggs come with antioxidants such as zeaxanthin and lutein, which can help maintain the eyes' proper health. Also, many people only consume the white portion of the egg. However, the majority of the nutrients are present in the egg yolk. So, it is essential to consume a complete egg.

Meat and Poultry

Meat is an important source of lean proteins and is also considered a staple on the keto diet. Fresh poultry and meat come with zero carbs and are also rich in B vitamins and various types of minerals, such as selenium, potassium, and zinc. Although processed meats, such as sausage and bacon, are permitted in the keto diet, they are not good for your heart's health. Excessive consumption of processed meats can also increase the overall risk of developing cancer. Try to limit processed meat as much as possible and opt for fresh meat and poultry.

Healthy Oils, Seeds, and Nuts

Seeds and nuts are rich in monounsaturated and polyunsaturated fats, protein, and fiber. They are also excessively low in net carb count. Coconut oil, along with olive oil, are the two recommended types of oils while being on a keto diet. Olive oil is rich in oleic acid. It can also be linked to lower risks of heart diseases. Coconut oil is a great source of saturated fats but also comes with MCTs or medium-chain triglycerides. It can readily help in increasing the overall production of ketones. MCTs can also help in improving the rate of metabolism and can promote weight loss and reduction of belly fat as well.

Unsweetened Tea and Coffee

Plain tea and coffee come with zero carbohydrates. So, they can be regarded as a perfect fit for the keto diet. It has been found that coffee can lower the overall risk of cardiovascular disease and type 2 diabetes. Tea comes with less caffeine and is high in antioxidants in comparison to coffee. It can help in weight loss, boost your immune system's functioning, and reduce stroke and heart attack risk.

Berries

Berries are a great source of antioxidants. They can help in protecting against diseases and can also reduce inflammation. They come with high fiber content and are low in carbs. Net carb count for half a cup of some common berries:

- **Raspberries:** Nine grams of net carbs

- **Blackberries:** Three grams of net carbs

- **Strawberries:** Three grams of net carbs

- **Blucberries:** Nine grams of net carbs

Chapter 4: Three-Week Keto Meal Plan

In this chapter, you will find a keto meal plan for twenty-one days, where your only aim will be to maintain the calorie count each day. The recipes are flexible, and you can replace any of the ingredients with ingredients of your choice to fit your liking. You can alter the recipes in this twenty-one days meal plan. Let us start with the breakfast plan first.

Breakfast Keto Meal Plan

Breakfast is most often regarded as an essential meal in a day. In this section, you will come across various breakfast recipes that can be altered in the twenty-one days meal challenge. Majority of the nutritionists suggest opting for a fulfilling breakfast so that you can stay full majority of the day.

Keto Fresh Spinach Frittata

Total Prep & Cooking Time: Forty-five minutes
Yields: Four servings
Nutrition Facts: Calories: 462.3 | Protein: 28.3g | Carbs: 3.4g| Fat: 47.6g | Fiber: 1.3g

Ingredients
- Five ounces of diced chorizo or bacon
- Two tbsps. of butter
- Eight ounces of spinach (fresh, chopped)

- Eight large eggs
- One cup of heavy cream (whipped)
- Five ounces of cheese (shredded)
- Pepper and salt (for seasoning)

Method:
1. Preheat your oven at one-hundred and seventy-five degrees Celsius. Grease a large baking dish with the help of cooking spray.

2. Heat the butter in an iron skillet. Add the chorizo. Fry until crispy. Add the chopped spinach. Cook for three minutes until wilted. Remove the skillet from the heat. Keep aside.

3. Whisk the cream along with the eggs in a large mixing bowl. Pour the egg mixture into the greased baking dish.

4. Add the spinach and bacon mix from the top. Add the cheese.

5. Bake for thirty minutes.

Baked Bacon Omelet

Total Prep & Cooking Time: Twenty-five minutes
Yields: Two servings
Nutrition Facts: Calories: 623.6 | Protein: 22.6g | Carbs: 2g| Fat: 71.3g | Fiber: 1.6g

Ingredients
- Four large eggs
- Five ounces of bacon (cubed)

- Three ounces of butter
- Two ounces of spinach (fresh)
- One tbsp. of chives (chopped)
- Pepper and salt (for seasoning)

Method:

1. Preheat your oven at two hundred degrees Celsius. Use butter for greasing a baking dish.

2. Heat remaining butter in an iron skillet. Fry the bacon cubes for one minute. Add the spinach and mix well.

3. Whisk the eggs in a medium-sized bowl. Combine the bacon spinach mixture. Mix properly.

4. Add pepper and salt. Add the chives and stir.

5. Pour the prepared mixture of egg into the greased baking dish.

6. Bake for twenty minutes.

7. Serve hot.

Keto Pancake With Whipped Cream and Berries

Total Prep & Cooking Time: Twenty-five minutes
Yields: Four servings
Nutrition Facts: Calories: 421.6 | Protein: 14.6g |
Carbs: 3.4g| Fat: 41.3g | Fiber: 3.2g

Ingredients
For the pancakes:
- Four large eggs
- Seven ounces of cottage cheese
- One tbsp. of ground psyllium husk powder
- Two ounces of butter

For the toppings:
- Two ounces of raspberries
- One cup of whipping cream

Method:
1. Combine together cottage cheese, eggs, and husk powder in a bowl. Mix well. Let the mixture sit for ten minutes.

2. Heat the butter in an iron skillet. Add half cup of the pancake mixture. Fry for four minutes on each side. Repeat with the remaining batter.

3. Add the whipping cream to a bowl. Keep whipping until it forms soft peaks.

4. Serve the pancakes in serving plates. Top with whipped cream and raspberries.

Coconut Porridge

Total Prep & Cooking Time: Ten minutes
Yields: Two servings
Nutrition Facts: Calories: 436.3 | Protein: 10.2g |
Carbs: 3.2g| Fat: 49.3g | Fiber: 5.2g

Ingredients

- One large egg (beaten)
- One tbsp. of coconut flour
- One pinch of ground psyllium husk powder
- Half tsp. of salt
- One ounce of butter
- Four tbsps. of coconut cream

Method:

1. Combine husk powder, coconut flour, salt, and egg in a medium-sized bowl.

2. Take a small pan. Heat the butter. Add the coconut cream and mix. Whisk in the mixture of egg slowly. Keep combining until the texture is thick and creamy.

3. Serve immediately with coconut cream.

Western Omelet

Total Prep & Cooking Time: Thirty minutes
Yields: Two servings
Nutrition Facts: Calories: 623.1 | Protein: 41.6g |
Carbs: 6.3g| Fat: 57.6g | Fiber: 1.1g

Ingredients
- Six large eggs
- Two tbsps. of sour cream
- Pepper and salt (for seasoning)
- Three ounces of cheese (shredded)
- Two ounces of butter
- Five ounces of smoked deli ham (diced)
- Half yellow onion (chopped)
- Half green bell pepper (chopped)

Method:
1. Whisk the cream along with the eggs in a bowl. Keep whisking until fluffy.

2. Add half of the cheese. Mix well.

3. Melt the butter in a large pan. Add the ham. Sauté for one minute. Add the onion along with the green bell pepper. Sauté for one minute.

4. Add the mixture of eggs. Keep cooking until the egg is set.

5. Lower the flame. Add remaining cheese from the top. Fold the omelet in half.

6. Serve hot.

Lunch Keto Meal Plan

In case you are confused about which recipes to include in your twenty-one days keto meal plan, this section has got all you need.

Asian Inspired Beef Salad

Total Prep & Cooking Time: Twenty-five minutes
Yields: Two servings
Nutrition Facts: Calories: 980.3 | Protein: 33.6g | Carbs: 5.7g| Fat: 98.6g | Fiber: 3.1g

Ingredients
For the sesame mayonnaise:
- Three-fourth cup of mayonnaise
- One tsp. of sesame oil
- Half tbsp. of lime juice
- Pepper and salt

For the beef:
- One tbsp. of each
  - Fish sauce
  - Olive oil
  - Ginger (grated)
- One tsp. of chili flakes
- Two-third pound of rib-eye steaks

For the salad:
- Three ounces of each
  - Lettuce
  - Cucumber
  - Cherry tomatoes

- Half red onion (sliced)
- Cilantro (chopped)
- One tsp. of sesame seeds
- Two scallions

Method:
1. Mix all the listed ingredients for the mayonnaise. Mix well. Keep aside.

2. Combine all the listed ingredients for the beef marinade in a large-sized bowl. Marinate the beef steaks for fifteen minutes.

3. Chop the veggies for the salad. Divide the salad among two plates.

4. Sear the steaks for five minutes on each side. Place the meat on a cutting board. Cut in thin slices.

5. Arrange the beef over the salad.

6. Serve immediately with a dollop of mayo mixture by the side.

Chicken Soup

Total Prep & Cooking Time: Thirty minutes
Yields: Eight servings
Nutrition Facts: Calories: 502.1 | Protein: 34.1g |
Carbs: 3.8g| Fat: 42.4g | Fiber: 1.2g

Ingredients
- Four ounces of butter
- Two tbsps. of dried onion (minced)
- Two stalks of celery (chopped)
- Six ounces of mushrooms (sliced)
- Two cloves of garlic (minced)
- Eight cups of chicken stock
- One carrot (sliced)
- Two tsps. of parsley (dried)
- One tsp. of salt
- One-fourth of black pepper (ground)
- One and a half rotisserie chicken (shredded)
- Five ounces of green cabbage (sliced)

Method:
1. Melt the butter in a deep pot.

2. Add celery, dried onion, garlic, and
   mushrooms. Sauté for four minutes.

3. Add carrot, chicken stock, parsley, pepper, and
   salt. Simmer for two minutes.

4. Add the chicken along with cabbage. Simmer
   for twelve minutes.

5. Serve hot.

Smoked Salmon Plate

Total Prep & Cooking Time: Five minutes
Yields: Two servings
Nutrition Facts: Calories: 963.2 | Protein: 36.3g |
Carbs: 1.1g| Fat: 98.7g | Fiber: 1.4g

Ingredients
- Three-fourth pound of smoked salmon
- One cup of mayonnaise
- Two ounces of baby spinach
- One tbsp. of olive oil
- Half lime
- Pepper and salt

Method:
1. Arrange spinach, salmon, lime wedge, and a dollop of mayo on serving plates.

2. Drizzle some olive oil from the top. Season with pepper and salt.

3. Serve immediately.

Keto Quesadillas

Total Prep & Cooking Time: Thirty minutes
Yields: Three servings
Nutrition Facts: Calories: 472.3 | Protein: 22.6g |
Carbs: 4.9g| Fat: 42.3g | Fiber: 3.2g

Ingredients
For the tortillas:
- Two large eggs
- Two eggs whites
- Six ounces of cream cheese
- Half tsp. of salt
- Two tsps. of ground psyllium husk powder
- One tbsp. of coconut flour

For the filling:
- One tbsp. of butter
- Five ounces of Mexican cheese blend
- One ounce of baby spinach

Method:
1. Preheat your oven at two hundred degrees Celsius.

2. Beat the egg whites and eggs in a bowl. Add the cream cheese. Blend using an electric mixer.

3. Mix salt, coconut flour, and husk powder in a bowl.

4. Add the mixture of flour in the egg mixture. Mix well.

5. Spread the batter on a greased baking sheet. Bake for ten minutes.

6. Cut the tortilla rectangle into six small pieces.

7. Heat the butter in a pan.

8. Add one tortilla. Sprinkle with spinach and cheese. Top with another tortilla.

9. Fry for one minute on each side.

Cauliflower Soup and Crispy Pancetta

Total Prep & Cooking Time: Twenty minutes
Yields: Six servings
Nutrition Facts: Calories: 536.4 | Protein: 11.3g |
Carbs: 5.6g| Fat: 54.6g | Fiber: 3.2g

Ingredients
- Four cups of chicken stock
- One pound of cauliflower
- One tbsp. of butter
- Seven ounces of cream cheese
- One and a half tbsp. of Dijon mustard
- Four ounces of butter
- Pepper and salt
- Seven ounces of pancetta (diced)
- One tsp. of paprika powder
- Three ounces of pecans

Method:
1. Cut the cauliflower into small florets.

2. Take a handful of the florets. Chop them into bite-size pieces.

3. Sauté pancetta and chopped florets in the butter for four minutes. Add paprika powder and nuts. Mix well.

4. Boil the florets of cauliflower in the stock. Add butter, mustard, and cream cheese.

5. Use an immersion blender for blending the
    soup. Blend until smooth. Add pepper and salt.

6. Divide the soup among serving bowls. Top with
    the fried mixture of pancetta.

7. Serve hot.

Dinner Keto Meal Plan

All the recipes that you will find in this section can help you bring about some serious changes in your health condition. Let's have a look at them.

Pesto Chicken Casserole With Cheese and Olives

Total Prep & Cooking Time: Forty-five minutes
Yields: Four servings
Nutrition Facts: Calories: 918.3 | Protein: 36.6g | Carbs: 5.7g| Fat: 94.3g | Fiber: 2.2g

Ingredients
- Two pounds of chicken breast
- Pepper and salt
- Two tbsps. of butter
- Five tbsps. of red pesto
- One and a half cup of whipping cream
- Three ounces of olives (pitted)
- Five ounces of feta cheese
- One clove of garlic (chopped)

Method:
1. Preheat your oven at two-hundred degrees Celsius.

2. Chop the chicken breast into bite-size cubes. Add pepper and salt.

3. Fry the chicken pieces in the butter.

4. Combine cream and red pesto in a bowl.

5. Arrange the cooked chicken pieces along with olives in a baking dish. Top with garlic and feta cheese. Add the mixture of pesto.

6. Bake for thirty minutes.

7. Serve hot.

Tortilla With Salsa and Ground Beef

Total Prep & Cooking Time: One hour and ten minutes
Yields: Four servings
Nutrition Facts: Calories: 820 | Protein: 41.3g | Carbs: 7.2g| Fat: 69.6g | Fiber: 12.3g

Ingredients
For the filling:
- Two tbsps. of olive oil
- One pound of beef (ground)
- Two tbsps. of tex-mex seasoning
- Half cup of water
- Pepper and salt

For the salsa:
- Two avocados (diced)
- One tomato (diced)
- Two tbsps. of lime juice
- One tbsp. of olive oil
- Half cup of cilantro (chopped)
- Pepper and salt

For serving:
- Six ounces of Mexican cheese (shredded)
- Three ounces of lettuce (shredded)
- Four low-carb tortillas

Method:
1. Take a large-sized non-stick pan and heat oil in it. Cook the beef for five minutes. Add water

and seasoning. Simmer for five minutes. Add pepper and salt.

2. Combine the salsa ingredients in a bowl.

3. Arrange beef and salsa on the tortillas. Top with cheese.

4. Serve with lettuce by the side.

Keto Pork Chops With Garlic Butter and Green Beans

Total Prep & Cooking Time: Thirty minutes
Yields: Four servings
Nutrition Facts: Calories: 730.3 | Protein: 37.6g |
Carbs: 5.8g| Fat: 63.6g | Fiber: 3.1g

Ingredients
For the garlic butter:
- Five ounces of butter
- Half tbsp. of garlic powder
- One tbsp. of each
  - Lemon juice
  - Parsley (dried)
- Pepper and salt

For the pork chops:
- Four pork chops
- Two ounces of butter
- One pound of green beans
- Pepper and salt

Method:
1. Combine the garlic butter ingredients in a bowl.

2. Use a sharp knife for making few cuts on the pork chops. Season with pepper and salt.

3. Melt the butter in an iron skillet. Add the chops. Fry for five minutes on each side. Remove the chops from the skillet.

4. Add the beans in the same skillet. Fry for two
    minutes. Season with pepper and salt.

5. Serve the chops with green beans and a
    spoonful of garlic butter on the top.

Fried Salmon With Cheese and Broccoli

Total Prep & Cooking Time: Thirty-five minutes
Yields: Four servings
Nutrition Facts: Calories: 682.6 | Protein: 45.9g |
Carbs: 5.9g| Fat: 51.6g | Fiber: 3.3g

Ingredients
- One pound of broccoli
- Three ounces of butter
- Pepper and salt
- Five ounces of cheddar cheese (grated)
- Two pounds of salmon
- One lime

Method:
1. Preheat your oven at two hundred degrees Celsius.

2. Chop the broccoli into small florets. Simmer the florets in salted water for five minutes. Drain the florets and keep aside.

3. Arrange the florets in a baking dish. Add pepper and butter.

4. Sprinkle grated cheese from the top. Bake for twenty minutes.

5. Season the fish with pepper and salt.

6. Heat butter in an iron skillet. Fry the fish on each side for four minutes.

7. Serve the fish with broccoli by the side. Garnish
   with lime wedges.

Rib-Eye Steak With Roasted Veggies

Total Prep & Cooking Time: Forty minutes
Yields: Four servings
Nutrition Facts: Calories: 797.6 | Protein: 42.1g |
Carbs: 9.8g| Fat: 66.3g | Fiber: 4.1g

Ingredients
- One pound of broccoli
- One whole garlic
- Ten ounces of cherry tomatoes
- Three tbsps. of olive oil
- One tbsp. of thyme (dried)
- Two pounds of rib-eye steaks
- Pepper and salt

For the anchovy butter:
- One ounce of anchovies
- Five ounces of butter
- One tbsp. of lemon juice
- Pepper and salt

Method:
1. Start with the anchovy butter by chopping the anchovy fillets. Combine with butter, pepper, lemon juice, and salt.

2. Preheat your oven at two hundred degrees Celsius.

3. Slice the broccoli into florets. Separate the cloves of garlic.

4. Grease a baking pan with butter. Add the veggies. Drizzle some olive oil from the top. Roast in the oven for fifteen minutes.

5. Season the steaks with pepper, salt, and add some olive oil.

6. Fry the steaks in an iron skillet for five minutes on each side.

7. Take out the veggie pan and make some room for the steaks.

8. Add the steaks in the pan along with the veggies.

9. Roast for fifteen minutes.

10. Serve with a spoonful of anchovy butter on the top.

Snacks Keto Meal Plan

Snacks form an important part of everyday meals. The aim is to satisfy your cravings without opting for something unhealthy. Here are some tasty keto snack recipes for you that you can make in no time.

Keto Bread Twists

Total Prep & Cooking Time: Forty minutes
Yields: Ten servings
Nutrition Facts: Calories: 210.3 | Protein: 8.6g |
Carbs: 1.1g| Fat: 18.3g | Fiber: 2.3g

Ingredients
- Half cup of almond flour
- One-fourth cup of coconut flour
- Half tsp. of salt
- One tsp. of baking powder
- One large egg (beaten)
- Two ounces of butter
- Seven ounces of cheese (shredded)
- One cup of green pesto
- One egg (for brushing)

Method:
1. Preheat your oven at one hundred and fifty degrees Celsius.

2. Mix all the dry listed ingredients along with the beaten egg.

3. Melt cheese and butter in a medium pot. Keep
    stirring until the batter becomes smooth.

4. Add the butter and cheese mixture to the dry
    ingredient mix. Mix well for making a firm
    dough.

5. Flatten the dough into a rectangle. Add green
    pesto on the top.

6. Cut the dough into strips of one-inch. Twist the
    strips. Arrange them on a baking pan. Brush
    the twisted strips with egg.

7. Bake for twenty minutes.

Burger Fat Bombs

Total Prep & Cooking Time: Thirty minutes
Yields: Ten servings
Nutrition Facts: Calories: 82.1 | Protein: 5g | Carbs: 0.2g| Fat: 7.2g | Fiber: 0.6g

Ingredients
- One pound of beef (ground)
- Cooking spray
- Half tsp. of garlic powder
- Kosher salt
- Black pepper (ground)
- Two tbsps. of butter (cut into twenty cubes)
- Two ounces of cheddar cheese (cut into twenty pieces)

Method:
1. Preheat your oven at one hundred and seventy degrees Celsius.

2. Use cooking spray for greasing a muffin tin.

3. Combine garlic powder, beef, pepper, and salt in a bowl.

4. Press one tsp. of the meat mixture into the base of each muffin cup. Add one cube of butter and top with one tsp. of meat. Add a piece of cheese on the top.

5. Bake for fifteen minutes.

6. Use a small knife for removing bombs.

7.   Serve hot.

Crab Avocado Boats

Total Prep & Cooking Time: Twenty minutes
Yields: Four servings
Nutrition Facts: Calories: 330.6 | Protein: 31.1g |
Carbs: 8.8g| Fat: 20.1g | Fiber: 5.3g

Ingredients

- Twelve ounces of crab meat
- One-third cup of Greek yogurt
- Half red onion (minced)
- Two tbsps. of chives (chopped)
- Three tbsps. of lemon juice
- Half tsp. of cayenne pepper
- Kosher salt
- One cup of cheddar cheese (shredded)
- Two avocados (halved, pitted)

Method:

1. Combine crab meat, yogurt, chives, red onion, cayenne, and lemon juice in a bowl. Add salt for seasoning.

2. Scoop out avocado pulp for making bowls. Add the scooped-out pulp in the mixture of crab.

3. Fill the avocado bowl with the mixture of crab. Add cheese from the top.

4. Broil for one minute.

**Keto Taquitos**

Total Prep & Cooking Time: Forty-five minutes
Yields: Six servings
Nutrition Facts: Calories: 229.6 | Protein: 18.2g |
Carbs: 2.1g| Fat: 19.8g | Fiber: 0.3g

Ingredients
- Two tbsps. of olive oil
- Half onion (chopped)
- Four garlic cloves (minced)
- One tsp. of each
    - Chili powder
    - Cumin (ground)
- Two cups of each
    - Chicken shredded
    - Monterey jack cheese (shredded)
    - Cheddar cheese (shredded)
- Two-third cup of red enchilada sauce
- Four tbsps. of cilantro (chopped)
- Kosher salt

Method:
1. Preheat your oven at one hundred and seventy degrees Celsius.

2. Use parchment paper for lining two baking sheets.

3. Heat oil in an iron skillet. Add chopped onion and garlic. Sauté for three minutes. Sprinkle the spices over the garlic-onion mixture. Keep stirring for two minutes. Now it is time to add

the chicken along with the enchilada sauce. Simmer the mixture for three minutes. Add cilantro. Keep aside.

4. Combine the cheeses in a bowl. Divide the cheese mixture into twelve equal three-inch piles on the baking sheets. Bake for ten minutes.

5. Let the taquito shells cool down for four minutes.

6. Add the chicken mixture in the shells and roll.

7. Serve immediately.

**Cheese, Ham, and Egg Roll-Ups**

Total Prep & Cooking Time: Thirty-five minutes
Yields: Ten servings
Nutrition Facts: Calories: 415.3 | Protein: 37.6g |
Carbs: 5.6g| Fat: 27.2g | Fiber: 1.2g

Ingredients

- Ten large eggs
- Two tsps. of garlic powder
- Kosher salt
- Black pepper (ground)
- Two tbsps. of butter
- Two cups of cheddar cheese (shredded)
- One cup of baby spinach
- Half cup of tomatoes (chopped)
- Two slices of ham

Method:

1. Beat the eggs with pepper, garlic powder, and salt in a mixing bowl.

2. Melt the butter in a skillet. Add the eggs. Scramble and cook for four minutes. Add the cheese, tomatoes, and spinach.

3. Place two ham slices on a cutting board. Add one tbsp. of the egg mixture. Roll the ham slices.

4. Arrange the rolled ham slices in a baking tray. Bake for five minutes.

5. Serve hot.

Chapter 5: Easy Keto Breakfast Recipes

Here are some tasty breakfast recipes for you with which you can start your day with a kick.

French Omelet

Total Prep & Cooking Time: Twenty minutes
Yields: Two servings
Nutrition Facts: Calories: 189 | Protein: 22.3g | Carbs: 3.6g| Fat: 10.9g | Fiber: 0.1g

Ingredients
- Two large eggs
- Four egg whites
- One-fourth cup of milk
- One-eighth tsp. of each
  - Pepper
  - Salt
- One cup of ham (cooked)
- One tbsp. of each
  - Green pepper (chopped)
  - Onion (chopped)
- Half cup of cheddar cheese (shredded)

Method:
1. Whisk the first five listed ingredients.

2. Use cooking spray for greasing a skillet. Place the skillet over medium flame. Add the mixture of eggs.

3. Cook for two minutes.

4. Top with the remaining ingredients. Fold the egg in half.

5. Cut the omelet in half. Serve immediately.

Sage Sausage Patty

Total Prep & Cooking Time: One hour and fifteen minutes
Yields: Eight servings
Nutrition Facts: Calories: 160.3 | Protein: 14.6g | Carbs: 1.2g| Fat: 12.3g | Fiber: 0.3g

Ingredients
- One pound of pork (ground)
- Three-fourth cup of cheddar cheese (ground)
- One-fourth cup of buttermilk
- One tbsp. of onion (chopped)
- Two tsps. of sage
- Three-fourth tsp. of each
  - Pepper
  - Salt
- Half tsp. of each
  - Oregano (dried)
  - Garlic powder

Method:
1. Combine the listed ingredients either in a bowl or in a food processor.

2. Shape the mixture into eight equal patties of half-inch. Refrigerate the patties for one hour.

3. Heat oil in an iron skillet. Cook the patties on each side for six minutes.

4. Serve hot.

Feta Frittata

Total Prep & Cooking Time: Thirty minutes
Yields: Two servings
Nutrition Facts: Calories: 205.3 | Protein: 19.3g |
Carbs: 6.7g| Fat: 12.5g | Fiber: 3.6g

Ingredients
- One green onion (sliced)
- One clove of garlic (minced)
- Two large eggs
- Half cup of egg substitute
- Four tbsps. of feta cheese (crumbled)
- One-third cup of plum tomato (chopped)
- Four slices of avocado (peeled)
- Two tbsps. of sour cream

Method:
1. Heat oil in an iron skillet. Add garlic and onion. Sauté for three minutes.

2. Combine egg substitute, eggs, and three tbsps. of feta cheese in a bowl. Add the mixture of eggs to the skillet.

3. Cook for six minutes.

4. Sprinkle remaining feta and tomato from the top.

5. Cover and cook for two minutes.

6. Let the egg stand for five minutes.

7. Serve with sour cream and avocado.

Ham Steak With Bacon, Mushrooms, and Gruyere

Total Prep & Cooking Time: Thirty-five minutes
Yields: Four servings
Nutrition Facts: Calories: 356.3 | Protein: 35.4g |
Carbs: 5.1g| Fat: 23.2g | Fiber: 1.1g

Ingredients
- Two tbsps. of butter
- Half pound of mushrooms (sliced)
- One shallot (chopped)
- Two cloves of garlic (minced)
- One-eighth tsp. of black pepper (ground)
- One boneless ham steak (cooked, cut in four equal pieces)
- One cup of gruyere cheese (shredded)
- Four strips of bacon (cooked, crumbled)
- One tbsp. of parsley (minced)

Method:
1. Heat butter in a large iron skillet. Add shallot and mushrooms. Cook the mixture for six minutes. Mix garlic and pepper. Sauté for two minutes. Keep aside.

2. Cook the ham in the same skillet. Add bacon and cheese. Cook for two minutes.

3. Serve the ham with the mushroom mixture from the top.

Mushroom-Mascarpone Frittata

Total Prep & Cooking Time: Forty-five minutes
Yields: Six servings
Nutrition Facts: Calories: 469.3 | Protein: 18.7g |
Carbs: 5.7g| Fat: 45.4g | Fiber: 1.6g

Ingredients
- Eight large eggs
- One-third cup of whipping cream
- Half cup of Romano cheese (grated)
- Two tsps. of salt
- Five tbsps. of olive oil
- Three-fourth pound of fresh mushrooms (sliced)
- One onion (sliced)
- Two tbsps. of basil (minced)
- Two cloves of garlic (minced)
- One-eighth tsp. of pepper
- Eight ounces of mascarpone cheese

Method:
1. Whisk together cream, eggs, one-fourth cup of Romano cheese, and salt in a bowl.

2. Heat two tbsps. of oil in a pan. Add mushrooms and onion. Sauté for two minutes. Add garlic, basil, along with pepper. Stir for one minute. Remove from heat. Add Romano cheese and mascarpone cheese.

3. Heat one tbsp. of oil in the same pan. Add half mixture of eggs in the pan. Keep cooking for

seven minutes. Repeat with the remaining egg mixture.

4. Place one egg frittata on a plate. Add the mixture of mushrooms. Spread properly.

5. Add the other layer of frittata.

6. Cut in wedges.

7. Serve immediately.

Broccoli Quiche Cups

Total Prep & Cooking Time: Twenty-five minutes
Yields: Six servings
Nutrition Facts: Calories: 292.3 | Protein: 17.6g |
Carbs: 3.6g| Fat: 25.4g | Fiber: 0.7g

Ingredients
- One cup of broccoli (chopped)
- One and a half cup of pepper jack cheese (shredded)
- Six large eggs
- Three-fourth cup of whipping cream
- Half cup of bacon bits
- One shallot (minced)
- One-fourth tsp. of each
  - Pepper
  - Salt

Method:
1. Preheat your oven at one-hundred and seventy degrees Celsius.

2. Divide the cheese and chopped broccoli among twelve greased muffin cups.

3. Combine the remaining ingredients in a bowl. Divide the prepared mixture among the cups.

4. Bake the quiche cups for twenty minutes.

5. Serve immediately.

Savory Chicken Sausage-Apple

Total Prep & Cooking Time: Twenty-five minutes
Yields: Four servings
Nutrition Facts: Calories: 93.6 | Protein: 9.9g | Carbs:
3.2g| Fat: 6.5g | Fiber: 1.2g

Ingredients
- One tart apple (peeled, diced)
- Two tsps. of poultry seasoning
- One tsp. of salt
- One-fourth tsp. of pepper
- One pound of chicken (ground)

Method:
1. Take a large bowl. Mix the first four
   ingredients. Crumble the chicken over the
   apple mixture. Combine well. Shape the
   mixture into eight equal patties of three-inch.

2. Heat oil in an iron skillet.

3. Cook the apple-chicken patties for six minutes
   on each side.

4. Serve hot.

Manchego and Shiitake Scramble

Total Prep & Cooking Time: Twenty-five minutes
Yields: Eight servings
Nutrition Facts: Calories: 270.6 | Protein: 12.1g |
Carbs: 3.4g| Fat: 23.6g | Fiber: 1.1g

Ingredients

- Two tbsps. of olive oil
- Half cup of each
    - Sweet red pepper (diced)
    - Onion (diced)
- Two cups of shiitake mushrooms (sliced)
- One tsp. of prepared horseradish
- Eight large eggs (beaten)
- One cup of each
    - Whipping cream
    - Manchego cheese (shredded)
- Half tsp. of each
    - Pepper (ground)
    - Kosher salt

Method:

1. Heat one tbsp. of oil in an iron skillet. Add red pepper and onion. Cook for three minutes. Cook the mixture for four minutes after adding the mushrooms along with horseradish. Stir for two minutes.

2. Whisk the remaining ingredients in a bowl with some olive oil. Pour the mixture into the skillet.

3. Cook and scramble the eggs for four minutes.

4. Serve hot.

**Three-Cheese Quiche**

Total Prep & Cooking Time: One hour and ten minutes
Yields: Six servings
Nutrition Facts: Calories: 448.3 | Protein: 21.2g | Carbs: 5.2g| Fat: 38.6g | Fiber: 0.2g

Ingredients
- Seven large eggs
- Five egg yolks
- One cup of each
  - Whipping cream
  - Half and half cream
  - Mozzarella cheese (shredded)
- Three-fourth cup of cheddar cheese (shredded)
- Half cup of Swiss cheese (shredded)
- Two tbsps. of sun-dried tomatoes
- One and half tsp. of seasoning blend
- One-fourth tsp. of basil (dried)

Method:
1. Preheat your oven at one hundred and fifty degrees Celsius.

2. Combine egg yolks, eggs, whipping cream, mozzarella cheese, half and half cream, half cup of cheddar cheese, tomatoes, Swiss cheese, basil, and seasoning blend in a greased pie dish. Sprinkle the remaining cheddar cheese from the top.

3. Bake for fifty minutes.

4. Let the quiche sit for ten minutes.

5. Cut in triangles and serve.

Breakfast Turkey Sausage

Total Prep & Cooking Time: Twenty minutes
Yields: Eight servings
Nutrition Facts: Calories: 87.6 | Protein: 11.3g | Carbs: 0.2g| Fat: 7.5g | Fiber: 0.1g

Ingredients

- One pound of lean turkey (ground)
- Three-fourth tsp. of salt
- Half tsp. of rubbed sage
- One-fourth tsp. of ginger (ground)
- One-third tsp. of pepper (ground)

Method:

1. Crumble the turkey meat in a large bowl. Add sage, salt, ginger, and pepper. Shape the mixture into eight equal patties of two-inch.

2. Grease an iron skillet with oil.

3. Add the patties. Cook for six minutes on each side.

<u>No-Bread Breakfast Sandwich</u>

Total Prep & Cooking Time: Fifteen minutes
Yields: Two servings
Nutrition Facts: Calories: 356.3 | Protein: 20.3g |
Carbs: 2.1g| Fat: 31.1g | Fiber: 0.2g

Ingredients
- Two tbsps. of butter
- Four large eggs
- Pepper and salt
- One ounce of deli ham (smoked)
- Two ounces of cheddar cheese (cut in slices)
- Few drops of Tabasco

Method:
1. Heat the butter in an iron skillet. Add the eggs. Fry each side for two minutes. Add pepper and salt.

2. Take a fried egg. Add ham and cheese. Top with another fried egg.

3. Repeat for the other fried eggs.

4. Place the sandwich in the pan for one minute.

5. Sprinkle some Tabasco from the top.

6. Serve hot.

Baked Eggs

Total Prep & Cooking Time: Twenty minutes
Yields: One serving
Nutrition Facts: Calories: 497.6 | Protein: 42.1g |
Carbs: 2.1g| Fat: 34.5g | Fiber: 0.3g

Ingredients
- Three ounces of beef (ground)
- Two large eggs
- Two ounces of cheese (shredded)

Method:
1. Preheat your oven at two hundred degrees Celsius.

2. Arrange the ground beef as the base in a baking dish.

3. Make two holes in the beef base. Crack the eggs in the holes.

4. Sprinkle cheese from the top.

5. Bake for fifteen minutes.

6. Let the baked eggs sit for five minutes.

Cured Salmon With Chives and Scrambled Eggs

Total Prep & Cooking Time: Fifteen minutes
Yields: Two servings
Nutrition Facts: Calories: 730.2 | Protein: 49.6g |
Carbs: 2.1g| Fat: 61.3g | Fiber: 0.1g

Ingredients
- Two large eggs
- Two tbsps. of butter
- One-fourth cup of whipping cream
- One tbsp. of chives (chopped)
- Two ounces of cured salmon
- Pepper and salt

Method:
1. Begin with whisking the eggs in a bowl.

2. Heat the butter in a pan. Add the eggs. Add the cream. Stir for three minutes.

3. Simmer for five minutes. Keep stirring for making the eggs creamy.

4. Add salt, chopped chives, and pepper.

5. Serve the eggs with cured salmon.

Eggs Benedict on Avocados

Total Prep & Cooking Time: Twenty minutes
Yields: Four servings
Nutrition Facts: Calories: 523.6 | Protein: 17.6g |
Carbs: 3.1g| Fat: 49.3g | Fiber: 7.1g

Ingredients
For the hollandaise:
- Three egg yolks
- One tbsp. of lemon juice
- Pepper and salt
- Eight tbsps. of butter (unsalted)

For the eggs:
- Two avocados (pitted, skinned)
- Four large eggs
- Five ounces of salmon (smoked)

Method:
1. Add the butter in a bowl. Microwave for twenty seconds.

2. Add lemon juice and egg yolks. Use a hand blender for properly blending the mixture. Keep blending until a white layer forms. Add pepper and salt. Blend for two minutes.

3. Boil water in a saucepan. Crack the eggs in a small cup. Crack one egg at a time. Slide the eggs gently into the water. Cook for four minutes.

4. Cut the avocados in half. Add an egg on top of each avocado slice. Add hollandaise sauce from the top.

5. Add smoked salmon by the side.

6. Serve immediately.

Keto Chaffles

Total Prep & Cooking Time: Ten minutes
Yields: Four servings
Nutrition Facts: Calories: 332.3 | Protein: 23.2g |
Carbs: 1.9g| Fat: 28.6g | Fiber: 0.2g

Ingredients
- One ounce of butter (melted)
- Four large eggs
- Eight ounces of mozzarella cheese (shredded)
- Four tbsps. of almond flour
- One pinch of salt

Method:
1. Preheat a waffle maker.

2. Mix all the ingredients that has been listed in a mixing bowl. Combine well.

3. Use butter for greasing the waffle maker.

4. Add one spoonful of the batter in the waffle maker. Close the waffle maker. Cook for six minutes.

5. Serve immediately with toppings of your choice.

Asparagus and Smoked Salmon Frittata

Total Prep & Cooking Time: Forty minutes
Yields: Four servings
Nutrition Facts: Calories: 511.3 | Protein: 28.9g |
Carbs: 3.4g| Fat: 44.3g | Fiber: 1.2g

Ingredients
- Eight large eggs
- One cup of whipping cream
- One tsp. of salt
- Half tsp. of pepper
- One and a half tsp. of dill (dried)
- Four ounces of mozzarella cheese (shredded)
- Two ounces of parmesan cheese (shredded)
- Half ounce of butter
- Three and a half ounces of smoked salmon
- Two and a half ounces of green asparagus

Method:
1. Preheat your oven at one hundred and fifty degrees Celsius.

2. Combine eggs, seasonings, cream, half of the mozzarella cheese, and parmesan cheese in a large bowl.

3. Use butter for greasing a baking dish.

4. Add chunks of smoked salmon all over the base of the baking dish.

5. Arrange the spears of asparagus over the base of salmon.

6. Pour the mixture of eggs over the asparagus. Sprinkle mozzarella from the top.

7. Bake the frittata for thirty minutes.

**Vegetable Keto Scramble**

Total Prep & Cooking Time: Twenty minutes
Yields: One serving
Nutrition Facts: Calories: 410.3 | Protein: 28.2g |
Carbs: 3.6g| Fat: 32.3g | Fiber: 1.1g

Ingredients
- One tbsp. of butter
- One ounce of mushrooms (sliced)
- Three large eggs
- One and a half ounces of red bell pepper (diced)
- Pepper and salt
- Half ounce of parmesan cheese (shredded)
- Half a scallion (chopped)

Method:
1. Melt the butter in an iron skillet. Add red peppers and mushrooms. Season with pepper and salt. Cook for four minutes.

2. Break the eggs into the skillet directly. Stir all the ingredients for combining.

3. Cook for four minutes. Keep stirring for keeping the eggs soft.

4. Serve with scallions and parmesan cheese from the top.

French Pancakes

Total Prep & Cooking Time: Fifteen minutes
Yields: Four servings
Nutrition Facts: Calories: 695 | Protein: 14.6g | Carbs: 3.3g| Fat: 67.8g | Fiber: 4.2g

Ingredients
- Eight large eggs
- Two cups of whipping cream
- Half cup of water
- One-fourth tsp. of salt
- Two tbsps. of psyllium husk powder
- Three ounces of butter

Method:
1. Combine cream, eggs, salt, and water in a bowl. Use a hand blender for proper mixing.

2. Add psyllium husk powder. Keep mixing. Let the batter rest for ten minutes.

3. Add butter in a pan. Fry the pancakes for four minutes on each side.

4. Serve hot.

Lettuce Wraps

Total Prep & Cooking Time: Twenty minutes
Yields: Two servings
Nutrition Facts: Calories: 580.6 | Protein: 12.3g |
Carbs: 3.9g| Fat: 57.6g | Fiber: 4.3g

Ingredients
- Six ounces of bacon slices
- Three tbsps. of mayonnaise
- Two ounces of lettuce
- Half an avocado
- One tomato (sliced)
- Pepper and salt

Method:
1. Fry the slices of bacon in an iron skillet. Fry for five minutes. Let the bacon slices sit for five minutes. Cut the strips in half.

2. Arrange the lettuce leaves on a cutting board. Squeeze lemon juice on the leaves. Add half slice of tomato, one slice of avocado, and three halves of bacon slices. Add pepper and salt.

3. Wrap the lettuce leaves.

4. Serve immediately.

Deviled Eggs

Total Prep & Cooking Time: Fifteen minutes
Yields: Four servings
Nutrition Facts: Calories: 167.3 | Protein: 7.6g | Carbs: 0.4g| Fat: 14.6g | Fiber: 0.2g

Ingredients
- Four large eggs
- One tsp. of Tabasco
- One-fourth cup of mayonnaise
- One pinch of herbal salt
- Eight shrimps (peeled, cooked)
- Dried dill

Method:
1. Boil the eggs in salted water. Boil for ten minutes.

2. Transfer the eggs to an ice bath. Let the eggs sit for two minutes. Peel the eggs.

3. Cut the eggs in half. Remove the yolks.

4. Arrange the eggs whites on a large plate.

5. Combine the yolks, mayonnaise, herbal salt, and Tabasco in one bowl. Use fork for mashing the ingredients.

6. Scoop two tsps. of the mixture of egg yolks into the egg whites. Top with the cooked shrimps.

7. Garnish with dill.

8. Serve immediately.

Keto Breakfast Cereal

Total Prep & Cooking Time: Forty minutes
Yields: Four servings
Nutrition Facts: Calories: 357.6 | Protein: 10.3g |
Carbs: 9.3g| Fat: 29.6g | Fiber: 5.6g

Ingredients

- One cup of each
    - Walnuts (chopped)
    - Almonds (chopped)
    - Coconut flakes
- One-fourth cup of sesame seeds
- Two tbsps. of each
    - Chia seeds
    - Flax seeds
- Half tsp. of clove (ground)
- Two tsps. of ground cinnamon
- One tsp. of vanilla extract
- One-third tsp. of kosher salt
- One large egg white
- One-fourth cup of coconut oil (melted)

Method:

1. Preheat your oven at one hundred and fifty degrees Celsius.

2. Use cooking spray for greasing a medium baking tray.

3. Combine walnuts, almonds, flax seeds, coconut flakes, sesame seeds, and chia seeds in a bowl.

Add cinnamon, cloves, salt, and vanilla extract. Mix well.

4. Beat the egg white in a small-sized bowl until foamy. Add it to the cereal mix.

5. Add the oil and mix.

6. Pour the cereal mix on the baking tray. Evenly spread out the cereal mix.

7. Bake for twenty minutes.

8. Let the cereal mix cool down completely and serve.

Breakfast Cups

Total Prep & Cooking Time: Forty minutes
Yields: Six servings
Nutrition Facts: Calories: 210.1 | Protein: 7.6g | Carbs: 1.2g| Fat: 53.4g | Fiber: 1.1g

Ingredients
- Two pounds of pork (ground)
- One tbsp. of thyme (chopped)
- Two cloves of garlic (minced)
- Half tsp. of each
    - Cumin (ground)
    - Paprika
- One tsp. of kosher salt
- Black pepper (ground)
- Three cups of spinach (chopped)
- One cup of white cheddar cheese (shredded)
- Twelve large eggs
- One tbsp. of chives (chopped)

Method:
1. Preheat your oven at two hundred degrees Celsius.

2. Combine thyme, pork, paprika, garlic, salt, and cumin in a bowl. Add pepper for seasoning.

3. Grease a muffin tin with cooking spray.

4. Add one handful of the pork mixture into each cup of the muffin tray. Press the mixture for

forming a cup. Arrange spinach and cheese among the meat cups.

5. Crack one egg over each cup. Season with pepper and salt.

6. Bake for twenty-five minutes.

7. Garnish with chopped chives.

8. Serve hot.

Omelet Stuffed Pepper

Total Prep & Cooking Time: One hour
Yields: Four servings
Nutrition Facts: Calories: 150.3 | Protein: 10.2g |
Carbs: 6.8g| Fat: 9.7g | Fiber: 1.9g

Ingredients

- Two bell peppers (halved, remove the seeds)
- Eight large eggs (beaten)
- One-fourth cup of milk
- Four bacon slices (cooked, crumbled)
- One cup of cheddar cheese (shredded)
- Two tbsps. of chives (chopped)
- Black pepper (ground)
- Kosher salt

Method:

1. Heat your oven at two hundred degrees Celsius.

2. Arrange the peppers in a baking dish with the cut side up.

3. Add some water in the dish. Bake for five minutes.

4. Combine milk and eggs in a bowl. Add cheese, bacon, and chives. Add pepper and salt for seasoning.

5. Divide the egg mixture among the peppers. Bake for forty minutes.

6. Garnish with chives.

7. Serve hot.

Brussels Sprouts Hash

Total Prep & Cooking Time: Forty minutes
Yields: Four servings
Nutrition Facts: Calories: 402.1 | Protein: 22.1g |
Carbs: 5.6g| Fat: 31.2g | Fiber: 4.6g

Ingredients

- Six bacon slices (cut in one-inch piece)
- Half onion (chopped)
- One pound of Brussels sprouts (trimmed, quartered)
- Kosher salt
- Black pepper (ground)
- One-fourth tsp. of red pepper flakes
- Two cloves of garlic (minced)
- Four large eggs

Method:

1. Cook the bacon pieces in an iron skillet until crispy. Keep aside.

2. Add Brussels sprouts and onion to the skillet. Add pepper, red pepper flakes, and salt. Cook for five minutes.

3. Add two tbsps. of water. Cover and cook for five minutes. Add the garlic. Cook for one minute.

4. Make four holes in the Brussels sprouts hash. Crack the eggs in the holes. Add pepper and salt.

5. Cover and cook for five minutes.

6. Garnish with cooked bits of bacon.

7. Serve hot.

Breakfast Stack

Total Prep & Cooking Time: Thirty minutes
Yields: Three servings
Nutrition Facts: Calories: 612.8 | Protein: 37.8g |
Carbs: 9.3g| Fat: 53.4g | Fiber: 6.8g

Ingredients

- Three patties of breakfast sausage
- One avocado (mashed)
- Black pepper (ground)
- Kosher salt
- Three large eggs
- Chopped chives (to garnish)

Method:

1. Prepare the breakfast sausage patties following the instructions on the box.

2. Add the mashed avocado on the sausage patties. Add pepper and salt.

3. Heat oil in a skillet. Crack the eggs. Season with pepper and salt. Cook for three minutes.

4. Add the eggs over the sausage patties.

5. Garnish with chopped chives.

6. Serve hot.

Cauliflower Benedict

Total Prep & Cooking Time: Thirty minutes
Yields: Two servings
Nutrition Facts: Calories: 269.3 | Protein: 17.6g |
Carbs: 6.3g| Fat: 17.3g | Fiber: 1.3g

Ingredients
For the patties:
- Half head of cauliflower
- One large egg
- Half tsp. of cornstarch
- One cup of cheddar cheese (shredded)
- Black pepper (ground)
- One tbsp. of olive oil

For the eggs:
- Two large eggs

For the sauce:
- Four large egg yolks
- Two tbsps. of lemon juice
- One tbsp. of butter (melted)
- Half tsp. of cayenne pepper
- Salt

For the assembly:
- Two slices of bacon (warmed)
- Paprika (to garnish)
- Chives (chopped, to garnish)

Method:

1. Grate the cauliflower. Combine eggs and grated
    cauliflower in a bowl. Add salt, cornstarch, and
    cheese. Mix well.

2. Make patties from the mixture.

3. Heat oil in an iron skillet. Add the patties. Cook
    for five minutes. Flip and cook for five minutes.

4. Start poaching the eggs in a large pot of hot
    water. Cook for three minutes.

5. Heat the egg yolks in a double boiler. Add the
    lemon juice and keep whisking. Add butter,
    salt, and cayenne. Mix well.

6. Serve the cauliflower patties and top with
    bacon, poached eggs, and sauce.

7. Garnish with chives and paprika.

Bacon Breakfast Tacos

Total Prep & Cooking Time: One hour
Yields: Four servings
Nutrition Facts: Calories: 395.6 | Protein: 24.2g |
Carbs: 4.1g| Fat: 31.1g | Fiber: 2.6g

Ingredients

- Sixteen bacon slices (halved)
- Black pepper (ground)
- Six large eggs
- One tbsp. of each
    - Butter
    - Whole milk
- Kosher salt
- Two tbsps. of chives (chopped)
- One-fourth cup of Monterey jack cheese
- One avocado (sliced)

Method:

1. For the taco shells: preheat your oven at two hundred degrees Celsius.

2. Line a baking sheet with the help of aluminum foil.

3. Prepare bacon weaves with eight halves of bacon for each. Make four weaves. Add pepper and salt. Bake for thirty minutes.

4. Trim the sides of the taco shells for making rounds.

5. Whisk milk and eggs in a bowl.

6. Melt the butter in an iron skillet. Add the egg mixture. Scramble the eggs for three minutes. Add pepper and salt.

7. Add scrambled eggs in the taco shells. Add avocado slices and sprinkle cheese from the top.

8. Serve immediately.

Loaded Cauliflower Bake

Total Prep & Cooking Time: One hour and fifteen minutes
Yields: Six servings
Nutrition Facts: Calories: 393.6 | Protein: 27.2g |
Carbs: 9.1g| Fat: 28.7g | Fiber: 3.2g

Ingredients
- One cauliflower
- Eight bacon slices (chopped)
- Ten large eggs
- Two cloves of garlic (minced)
- One cup of milk
- Two tsps. of paprika
- Kosher salt
- Two cups of cheddar cheese (shredded)
- Black pepper (ground)
- Two green onions (sliced)

Method:
1. Preheat your oven at one hundred and fifty degrees Celsius.

2. Grate the cauliflower.

3. Cook the bacon slices in an iron skillet for eight minutes.

4. Combine milk, eggs, paprika, and garlic in a bowl. Add pepper and salt.

5. Transfer grated cauliflower to a large baking dish. Top with cheddar cheese, green onions, and bacon. Pour over the mixture of eggs.

6. Bake for forty minutes.

7. Serve hot.

Chapter 6: Easy Keto Lunch Recipes

In this chapter, you will find some tasty keto lunch recipes that you can include in your diet plan without any worries. Let's have a look at them.

Turkey and Cream Cheese Sauce

Total Prep & Cooking Time: Twenty-five minutes
Yields: Five servings
Nutrition Facts: Calories: 810.3 | Protein: 47.6g | Carbs: 6.9g| Fat: 68.6g | Fiber: 0.6g

Ingredients

- Two tbsps. of butter
- Two pounds of turkey breast
- Two cups of whipping cream
- Seven ounces of cream cheese
- One tbsp. of tamari soy sauce
- Pepper and salt
- One and a half ounces of small capers

Method:

1. Preheat your oven at one hundred and seventy degrees Celsius.

2. Melt half butter in an iron skillet.

3. Season the breast of turkey with pepper and salt. Fry for five minutes.

4. Place the skillet in the oven. Bake for ten minutes.

5. Add the drippings of turkey in a pan. Add cream cheese and whipping cream. Simmer the mixture. Add pepper, soy sauce, and salt.

6. Sauté the small capers in remaining butter.

7. Slice the turkey.

8. Serve with fried capers and cream cheese sauce.

Baked Salmon and Pesto

Total Prep & Cooking Time: Twenty minutes
Yields: Four servings
Nutrition Facts: Calories: 1010.2 | Protein: 51.6g |
Carbs: 3.1g| Fat: 87.6g | Fiber: 0.7g

Ingredients

For the green sauce:
- Four tbsps. of green pesto
- One cup of mayonnaise
- Half cup of Greek yogurt
- Pepper and salt

For the salmon:
- Two pounds of salmon
- Four tbsps. of green pesto
- Pepper and salt

Method:

1. Place the fillets of salmon on a greased baking dish with the skin side down. Add pesto on top. Add pepper and salt.

2. Bake at two hundred degrees Celsius for thirty minutes.

3. Combine all the listed ingredients for the green sauce in a bowl.

4. Serve the baked salmon with green sauce on top.

Keto Chicken With Butter and Lemon

Total Prep & Cooking Time: Two hours and ten minutes
Yields: Four servings
Nutrition Facts: Calories: 980.3 | Protein: 57.2g | Carbs: 0.4g | Fat: 81.3g | Fiber: 0.1g

Ingredients

- Three pounds of a whole chicken
- Pepper and salt
- Two tsps. of barbecue seasoning rub (dry)
- Five ounces of butter (sliced)
- One lemon (cut in wedges)
- Two onions (cut in wedges)
- One-fourth cup of water
- One tsp. of butter (to grease)

Method:

1. Preheat your oven at one hundred and seventy degrees Celsius.

2. Use butter for greasing a deep baking dish.

3. Season the chicken with pepper, salt, and barbecue rub. Place the chicken in the greased baking dish.

4. Arrange lemon wedges and onions surrounding the chicken. Add slices of butter on the chicken.

5. Bake for one hour and thirty minutes. Make sure you baste the whole chicken with the drippings occasionally.

6. Cut the chicken in pieces.

7. Serve hot.

Garlic Chicken

Total Prep & Cooking Time: One hour and ten minutes
Yields: Four servings
Nutrition Facts: Calories: 540.3 | Protein: 41.3g | Carbs: 3.1g| Fat: 38.6g | Fiber: 1.6g

Ingredients
- Two ounces of butter
- Two pounds of chicken drumsticks
- Pepper and salt
- One lemon (juiced)
- Two tbsps. of olive oil
- Seven cloves of garlic (sliced)
- Half cup of parsley (chopped)

Method:
1. Preheat your oven at two hundred and fifty degrees Celsius.

2. Arrange the pieces of chicken in a greased baking dish. Add pepper and salt.

3. Add olive oil along with lemon juice over the chicken. Sprinkle parsley and garlic on top.

4. Bake for forty minutes.

5. Serve hot.

Salmon Skewers Wrapped With Prosciutto

Total Prep & Cooking Time: Thirty-five minutes
Yields: Four servings
Nutrition Facts: Calories: 670.5 | Protein: 27.2g |
Carbs: 1.2g| Fat: 61.6g | Fiber: 0.3g

Ingredients

- One-fourth cup of basil (chopped)
- One pound of salmon
- One pinch of black pepper (ground)
- Four ounces of prosciutto (sliced)
- One tbsp. of olive oil
- Eight skewers (wooden)

Method:

1. Start by soaking the skewers in a bowl of water.

2. Cut the salmon fillets length-wise. Thread the salmon on the soaked skewers.

3. Coat the skewers in pepper and basil.

4. Wrap the slices of prosciutto all around the salmon.

5. Heat oil in a grill pan. Grill the skewers for four minutes.

6. Serve hot.

Buffalo Drumsticks and Chili Aioli

Total Prep & Cooking Time: Fifty minutes
Yields: Four servings
Nutrition Facts: Calories: 567.8 | Protein: 41.3g |
Carbs: 2.2g| Fat: 43.2g | Fiber: 1.1g

Ingredients
For the chili aioli:
- Half cup of mayonnaise
- One tbsp. of smoked paprika powder
- One clove of garlic (minced)

For the chicken:
- Two pounds of chicken drumsticks
- Two tbsps. of each
  - White wine vinegar
  - Olive oil
- One tbsp. of tomato paste
- One tsp. of each
  - Salt
  - Paprika powder
  - Tabasco

Method:
1. Preheat your oven at two hundred degrees Celsius.

2. Combine the listed marinade ingredients. Marinate the chicken drumsticks for ten minutes.

3. Coat a baking tray with oil.

4. Arrange the chicken drumsticks in the tray.
    Bake for forty minutes.

5. Combine the listed ingredients for the chili aioli
    in a bowl.

6. Serve the drumsticks with chili aioli by the side.

Slow Cooked Roasted Pork and Creamy Gravy

Total Prep & Cooking Time: Eight hours and forty minutes
Yields: Six servings
Nutrition Facts: Calories: 586.9 | Protein: 27.9g | Carbs: 2.6g| Fat: 50.3g | Fiber: 1.5g

Ingredients
For the creamy gravy:
- Two cups of whipping cream
- Roast juice

For the pork:
- Two pounds of pork roast
- Half tbsp. of salt
- One bay leaf
- Five black peppercorns
- Three cups of water
- Two tsps. of thyme (dried)
- Two cloves of garlic
- Two ounces of ginger
- One tbsp. of each
    - Paprika powder
    - Olive oil
- One-third tsp. of black pepper (ground)

Method:
1. Preheat your oven at one hundred degrees Celsius.

2. Add the meat in a baking dish. Add salt. Add water for covering one-third of the meat. Add peppercorns, thyme, and bay leaf. Place the meat in the oven for eight hours. Cover the dish with aluminum foil.

3. Take out the meat from the oven. Reserve the juices from the dish.

4. Increase the temperature of the oven to two hundred degrees Celsius.

5. Grate ginger and garlic in a bowl. Add pepper, herbs, and oil. Rub the herb mixture on the meat.

6. Roast the meat for fifteen minutes.

7. Cut the roasted meat in slices.

8. Strain the meat juices in a bowl. Boil for reducing it by half.

9. Add the cream. Mix well. Simmer for twenty minutes.

10. Serve the roasted pork with creamy gravy from the top.

Bacon-Wrapped Meatloaf

Total Prep & Cooking Time: One hour twenty-five minutes
Yields: Four servings
Nutrition Facts: Calories: 1020.3 | Protein: 46.7g | Carbs: 5.6g| Fat: 88.9g | Fiber: 1.2g

Ingredients
For the meatloaf:
- Two tbsps. of butter
- One onion (chopped)
- Two pounds of beef (ground)
- Half cup of whipping cream
- Two ounces of cheese (shredded)
- One large egg (beaten)
- One tbsp. of oregano (dried)
- One tsp. of salt
- Half tsp. of black pepper (ground)
- Seven ounces of bacon (sliced)

For the gravy:
- One and a half cup of whipping cream
- Half tbsp. of tamari soy sauce

Method:
1. Preheat your oven at two hundred degrees Celsius.

2. Melt the butter in a pan. Add the onion. Cook for four minutes. Keep aside.

3. Combine onion, ground meat, and the remaining ingredients in a large bowl. Do not mix the bacon.

4. Make a firm loaf. Add the meatloaf in an oil-greased baking dish. Use bacon strips for wrapping the loaf.

5. Bake the meatloaf for forty-five minutes.

6. Add the juices from the baking dish in a pan. Add the cream and boil. Simmer for ten minutes. Add the soy sauce.

7. Slice the meatloaf. Serve with gravy from the top.

Lamb Chops and Herb Butter

Total Prep & Cooking Time: Fifteen minutes
Yields: Four servings
Nutrition Facts: Calories: 722.3 | Protein: 42.3g |
Carbs: 0.4g| Fat: 61.5g | Fiber: 0.4g

Ingredients

- Eight lamb chops
- One tbsp. of each
    - Olive oil
    - Butter
- Pepper and salt

For the herb butter:

- Five ounces of butter
- One clove of garlic (mashed)
- Half tbsp. of garlic powder
- Four tbsps. of parsley (chopped)
- One tsp. of lemon juice
- One-third tsp. of salt

Method:

1. Season the lamb chops with pepper and salt.

2. Heat olive oil and butter in an iron skillet. Add the lamb chops. Fry for four minutes.

3. Combine all the listed ingredients for the herb butter in a bowl. Let the herb butter sit for fifteen minutes.

4. Serve the lamb chops with herb butter by the
    side.

<u>Crispy Cuban Pork Roast</u>

Total Prep & Cooking Time: Nine hours and twenty minutes
Yields: Six servings
Nutrition Facts: Calories: 910.3 | Protein: 58.3g | Carbs: 5.3g| Fat: 69.6g | Fiber: 2.2g

Ingredients
- Five pounds of pork shoulder
- Four tsps. of salt
- Two tsps. of cumin (ground)
- One tsp. of black pepper (ground)
- Two tbsps. of oregano
- One red onion (diced)
- Four cloves of garlic
- One orange (juiced)
- Two lemons (juiced)
- One-fourth cup of olive oil

Method:
1. Rub the pork shoulder with salt. Place the meat in a bowl.

2. Mix all the remaining ingredients of the marinade in a blender.

3. Pour the marinade all over the meat. Marinate in the refrigerator for eight hours.

4. Place the meat in a pressure cooker. Add the marinade.

5. Cook for forty minutes.

6. Preheat your oven at two hundred degrees Celsius.

7. Roast the pork for thirty minutes.

8. Collect the juice from the pressure cooker and boil. Simmer for twenty minutes.

9. Shred the meat using a fork into large chunks.

10. Pour the juice all over the meat.

11. Serve immediately.

Keto Barbecued Ribs

Total Prep & Cooking Time: One hour and forty minutes
Yields: Four servings
Nutrition Facts: Calories: 980.3 | Protein: 54.3g | Carbs: 5.8g| Fat: 80.2g | Fiber: 4.6g

Ingredients

- One-fourth cup of Dijon mustard
- Two tbsps. of each
    - Cider vinegar
    - Butter
    - Salt
- Three pounds of spare ribs
- Four tbsps. of paprika powder
- Half tbsp. of chili powder
- One and a half tbsp. of garlic powder
- Two tsps. of each
    - Onion powder
    - Cumin (ground)
- Two and a half tbsp. of black pepper (ground)

Method:

1. Preheat a grill for thirty minutes.

2. For preparing the wet base, mix vinegar and Dijon mustard in a bowl. Add the ribs and coat well.

3. For preparing the dry rub, mix all the listed spices. Rub the mix all over the ribs. Reserve some for later use.

4. Arrange the coated ribs on an aluminum foil. Add some butter over the ribs.

5. Take the sides of the foil and seal them. Repeat with another foil from outside.

6. Place the wrapped ribs on the preheated grill for one hour. Close the lid.

7. Open the foil and arrange the ribs on a cutting board. Sprinkle reserved spice mix. Return the ribs to the grill. Grill for ten minutes.

8. Serve hot.

**Turkey Burgers and Tomato Butter**

Total Prep & Cooking Time: Forty minutes
Yields: Four servings
Nutrition Facts: Calories: 830.4 | Protein: 33.6g |
Carbs: 6.7g| Fat: 71.5g | Fiber: 5.1g

Ingredients
For the chicken patties:
- Two pounds of chicken (ground)
- One large egg
- Half onion (chopped)
- One tsp. of salt
- Half tsp. of black pepper (ground)
- One and a half tsp. of thyme (dried)
- Two ounces of butter

For the fried cabbage:
- Two pounds of green cabbage
- Three ounces of butter
- One tsp. of salt
- Half tsp. of black pepper (ground)

For the tomato butter:
- Four ounces of butter
- One tbsp. of tomato paste
- One tsp. of red wine vinegar
- Pepper and salt

Method:
1. Preheat your oven at one hundred degrees Celsius.

2. Combine the listed ingredients for the patties in a large bowl.

3. Shape the mixture into patties using your hands.

4. Heat butter in an iron skillet. Fry the chicken patties for five minutes on each side.

5. Place the patties in the oven for keeping them warm.

6. Heat butter in a pan. Add the cabbage. Add pepper and salt. Fry for five minutes.

7. Whip the ingredients for the tomato butter in a bowl. Use an electric mixer for even mixing.

8. Arrange the turkey patties on a serving plate. Top with fried cabbage. Serve with a dollop of tomato butter from the top.

Keto Hamburger

Total Prep & Cooking Time: One hour and ten
minutes
Yields: Four servings
Nutrition Facts: Calories: 1070.3 | Protein: 53.4g |
Carbs: 6.1g| Fat: 85.3g | Fiber: 12.3g

Ingredients
For the burger buns:
- Two cups of almond flour
- Five tbsps. of ground psyllium husk powder
- Two tsps. of baking powder
- One tsp. of salt
- One and a half cup of water
- Two tsps. of cider vinegar
- Three egg whites
- One tbsp. of sesame seeds

For the hamburger:
- Two pounds of beef (ground)
- One ounce of olive oil
- Pepper and salt
- One and a half ounce of lettuce (shredded)
- One tomato (sliced)
- One red onion (sliced)
- Half cup of mayonnaise
- Five ounces of bacon

Method:
1. Preheat your oven at one hundred and fifty
   degrees Celsius.

2. Mix the listed dry ingredients for the buns in a bowl.

3. Boil the water.

4. Add egg whites, water, and vinegar to the dry mix. Mix well.

5. Make individual pieces of buns with your hands. Sprinkle some sesame seeds on the top.

6. Bake for sixty minutes

7. Fry the slices of bacon in an iron skillet. Keep aside.

8. Mix beef, pepper, and salt in a bowl. Make patties using your hands.

9. Heat a grill pan. Brush the pan with some oil. Grill the beef patties for five minutes on each side.

10. Combine mayonnaise and lettuce in a bowl.

11. Cut the buns in half. Add beef patty, lettuce mix, onion slice, and tomato slice in one half of a bun. Top with bacon slices. Add the other half of the bun.

12. Serve immediately.

Chicken Wings and Blue Cheese Dressing

Total Prep & Cooking Time: One hour and thirty minutes
Yields: Four servings
Nutrition Facts: Calories: 839.3 | Protein: 51.2g | Carbs: 2.9g| Fat: 67.8g | Fiber: 0.2g

Ingredients
- One-third cup of mayonnaise
- One-fourth cup of sour cream
- Three tsps. of lemon juice
- One-fourth tsp. of each
  - Salt
  - Garlic powder
- Half cup of whipping cream
- Three ounces of blue cheese (crumbled)

For the chicken wings:
- Two pounds of chicken wings
- Two tbsps. of olive oil
- One-fourth tsp. of garlic powder
- One clove of garlic (minced)
- One-third tsp. of black pepper (ground)
- One tsp. of salt
- Two ounces of parmesan cheese (grated)

Method:
1. Mix all the blue cheese dressing ingredients in a bowl. Chill in the refrigerator for forty minutes.

2. Combine the chicken with olive oil and spices.
    Marinate for thirty minutes in the refrigerator.

3. Bake in the oven for twenty-five minutes.

4. Toss the chicken wings with parmesan cheese
    in a bowl.

5. Serve the chicken wings with blue cheese
    dressing by the side.

Salmon Burgers With Lemon Butter and Mash

Total Prep & Cooking Time: Thirty minutes
Yields: Four servings
Nutrition Facts: Calories: 1025.3 | Protein: 44.5g | Carbs: 6.8g| Fat: 90.1g | Fiber: 3.1g

Ingredients
For the salmon burgers:
- Two pounds of salmon
- One large egg
- Half yellow onion
- One tsp. of salt
- Half tsp. of black pepper (ground)
- Two ounces of butter

For the green mash:
- One pound of broccoli
- Five ounces of butter
- Two ounces of parmesan cheese (grated)
- Pepper and salt

For the lemon butter:
- Four ounces of butter
- Two tbsps. of lemon juice
- Pepper and salt

Method:
1. Preheat your oven at one hundred degrees Celsius.

2. Cut the salmon into small pieces. Combine all the burger ingredients along with the fish in a blender. Pulse for thirty seconds.

3. Make eight patties using your hands.

4. Heat butter in an iron skillet. Fry the burgers for five minutes on all sides.

5. Cut the broccoli into small florets. Boil water along with some salt in a pot. Add the broccoli. Cook for three to four minutes. Drain the water.

6. Add parmesan cheese and butter. Use an immersion blender for blending the ingredients. Add pepper and salt.

7. Combine lemon juice with butter, pepper, and salt. Beat using an electric beater.

8. Serve the salmon burgers with a dollop of lemon butter on the top and green mash by the side.

Cheeseburger

Total Prep & Cooking Time: Thirty-five minutes
Yields: Four servings
Nutrition Facts: Calories: 1190.3 | Protein: 53.1g | Carbs: 6.6g| Fat: 105.2g | Fiber: 6.3g

Ingredients
For the salsa:
- Two tomatoes (chopped)
- Two scallions (chopped)
- One avocado (chopped)
- One tbsp. of olive oil
- Salt
- Cilantro (chopped)

For the burgers:
- Two pounds of beef (ground)
- Seven ounces of cheese (shredded)
- Two tsps. of each
  - Paprika powder
  - Garlic powder
  - Onion powder
- Two tbsps. of oregano (chopped)
- Two ounces of butter
- Pepper and salt

For the toppings:
- Five ounces of lettuce
- Three-fourth cup of mayonnaise
- Five ounces of bacon (cooked, crumbled)
- Four tbsps. of pickled jalapenos (chopped)

- Three ounces of dill pickles (sliced)
- Five tbsps. of Dijon mustard

Method:
1. Combine the salsa ingredients. Keep aside.

2. Combine the ingredients that have been listed for the burger in a large bowl. Make four patties using your hands.

3. Heat butter in an iron skillet. Add the burgers. Fry for five minutes.

4. Serve the burgers on lettuce leaves. Top with bacon, mayonnaise, dill pickle, jalapenos, and mustard. Add salsa from the top.

Beef Tenderloin With Pepper Crust and Herbed Steak Sauce

Total Prep & Cooking Time: One hour and ten minutes
Yields: Four servings
Nutrition Facts: Calories: 11127.3 | Protein: 45.4g | Carbs: 3.9g| Fat: 108.9g | Fiber: 2.2g

Ingredients
For the beef:
- Two pounds of beef tenderloin
- Two tsps. of garlic powder
- Three tsps. of onion powder
- One tbsp. of black pepper (ground coarsely)
- Half tsp. of salt
- Two tbsps. of olive oil

For the sauce:
- Nine ounces of butter
- One tbsp. of each
  - Garlic cloves (minced)
  - Lemon juice
  - Dijon mustard
  - Chives (chopped)
- Two tbsps. of parsley (chopped)
- One tsp. of each
  - Oregano (dried)
  - Thyme (dried)
- Pepper and salt

For serving:

- Four ounces of leafy greens

Method:
1. Combine all the listed spice rub ingredients in a bowl. Sprinkle the mix of spices in a shallow dish. Roll the meat until it gets coated properly.

2. Let the beef sit for thirty minutes.

3. Heat a large grill pan. Add some olive oil. Place the beef and sear for seven minutes on all sides.

4. Slice the beef.

5. Add all the listed ingredients for the sauce in a pot. Mix well and simmer for ten minutes.

6. Serve the beef tenderloin slices in a serving plate with leafy greens. Drizzle the sauce on top.

Beetroot Cured Salmon and Dill Oil

Total Prep & Cooking Time: Twenty-four hours and ten minutes
Yields: Four servings
Nutrition Facts: Calories: 510.2 | Protein: 23.6g | Carbs: 4.2g| Fat: 43.2g | Fiber: 2.2g

Ingredients
- One large beet
- Two tbsps. of salt
- Five white peppercorns
- One lime (zested)
- One pound of salmon

For the dill oil:
- Half cup of dill (chopped)
- One tbsp. of spinach
- One-third cup of olive oil
- Pepper and salt

For serving:
- Two ounces of daikon (sliced)
- One pound of lettuce

Method:
1. Grate the beetroot and add it in a bowl. Ground the peppercorns and add it in the bowl. Add lime zest and salt.

2. Arrange the salmon on a large plate with the skin side down. Rub the beetroot mixture on

the flesh side. Cover using a cling film. Leave the salmon sit in the refrigerator for one day.

3. Combine spinach and dill in a bowl using a hand blender. Add pepper, salt, and oil.

4. Take out the salmon. Use a brush for removing the beetroot cure.

5. Cut the salmon into thin slices.

6. Serve with lettuce and chopped daikon. Drizzle dill oil from the top.

Zucchini Pizza Boats

Total Prep & Cooking Time: Forty minutes
Yields: Four servings
Nutrition Facts: Calories: 690.3 | Protein: 28.6g |
Carbs: 5.2g| Fat: 63.2g | Fiber: 2.6g

Ingredients

- One zucchini
- Two cloves of garlic (minced)
- Four tbsps. of olive oil
- Two ounces of baby spinach
- Pepper and salt
- Two tbsps. of marinara sauce
- Eight ounces of goat cheese

Method:

1. Preheat your oven at one hundred and ninety degrees Celsius.

2. Slice the zucchini lengthwise in half. Scrape out the seeds using a spoon.

3. Arrange the zucchini boats on a baking tray.

4. Take a non-stick pan and heat oil in it. Sauté the garlic for three minutes. Add zucchini seeds and spinach. Add pepper and salt.

5. Add marinara sauce over the boats. Top with the spinach mixture. Add cheese on top of the boats.

6. Bake the zucchini boats for twenty minutes.

7. Serve immediately.

Shrimp Salad With Bacon Fat Dressing

Total Prep & Cooking Time: Twenty minutes
Yields: Four servings
Nutrition Facts: Calories: 450.6 | Protein: 20.3g |
Carbs: 1.9g| Fat: 39.6g | Fiber: 1.1g

Ingredients

For the shrimp salad:

- Six ounces of spinach
- Two ounces of bacon (chopped)
- Two boiled eggs (chopped)
- One pound of shrimp (peeled)
- One tbsp. of butter
- One ounce of parmesan cheese (grated)

For the bacon fat dressing:

- Half cup of bacon fat
- One-fourth cup of apple cider vinegar
- One tbsp. of Dijon mustard
- Pepper and salt

Method:

1. Divide the spinach leaves evenly among serving plates after proper cleaning.

2. Heat oil in an iron skillet. Fry the bacon until crispy.

3. Arrange chopped eggs and bacon over the spinach bed.

4. Heat butter in the same skillet. Add the shrimps. Sauté for five minutes.

5. Divide the cooked shrimps among the plates. Top with cheese.

6. Melt the bacon fat in a small pan. Add the remaining ingredients. Mix well.

7. Drizzle bacon fat dressing on the salad.

8. Serve immediately.

Seafood Salad and Avocado

Total Prep & Cooking Time: Twenty minutes
Yields: Six servings
Nutrition Facts: Calories: 432.8 | Protein: 26.9g |
Carbs: 2.6g| Fat: 35.4g | Fiber: 2.1g

Ingredients

- Two tbsps. of lime juice
- Half cup of each
  - Sour cream
  - Mayonnaise
- One clove of garlic (minced)
- One tsp. of salt
- One ounce of red onion (minced)
- One-fourth tsp. of white pepper
- One pound of salmon (cooked, chopped in bite-size pieces)
- Half pound of shrimp (cooked, chopped)
- One avocado (chopped)
- Two ounces of cucumber (chopped)
- Three ounces of tomatoes (chopped)

Method:

1. Combine mayonnaise, lime juice, garlic, sour cream, pepper, onion, and salt in a mixing bowl.

2. Toss together shrimp, cucumber, salmon, tomato, and avocado in another bowl.

3. Add the mayo dressing over the mixture of veggies and seafood. Toss well.

4. Chill in the refrigerator for ten minutes.

Chorizo With Green Cabbage Cream

Total Prep & Cooking Time: Twenty-five minutes
Yields: Six servings
Nutrition Facts: Calories: 1176.3 | Protein: 47.2g |
Carbs: 8.2g| Fat: 112.5g | Fiber: 5.2g

Ingredients
For the green cabbage:
- Two pounds of green cabbage
- Two ounces of butter
- Two cups of whipping cream
- Pepper and salt
- Half cup of parsley (chopped)
- Half tbsp. of lemon zest

For the chorizo:
- Two pounds of chorizo
- Two tbsps. of butter

Method:
1. Heat butter in an iron skillet. Add the chorizo. Fry for four minutes.

2. Add the cabbage in a food processor. Shred the cabbage properly.

3. Add remaining butter in the skillet. Add the cabbage. Sauté for five minutes.

4. Add cream, pepper, and salt. Simmer for five minutes.

5. Add lemon zest and parsley. Simmer for two minutes.

6. Serve the chorizo with creamy green cabbage by the side.

Chapter 7: Easy Keto Dinner Recipes

The main motive of a keto diet is to take care of the carb consumption. This chapter is all about some exciting and tasty keto dinner recipes that are low in carbs.

Tex-Mex Casserole

Total Prep & Cooking Time: Forty minutes
Yields: Four servings
Nutrition Facts: Calories: 750.2 | Protein: 48.6g | Carbs: 7.5g| Fat: 55.7g | Fiber: 4.2g

Ingredients

- Two pounds of beef (ground)
- Two ounces of butter
- Three tbsps. of Tex-Mex seasoning
- Seven ounces of tomatoes (crushed)
- Three ounces of pickled jalapenos
- Six ounces of cheese (shredded)

For serving:

- Three-fourth cup of sour cream
- One scallion (chopped)
- Five ounces of leafy greens
- One cup of guacamole

Method:

1. Preheat your oven at two hundred degrees Celsius.

2. Heat butter in an iron skillet. Add the ground beef. Fry for five minutes.

3. Add the crushed tomatoes along with the seasoning. Simmer for five minutes.

4. Pour the beef mixture in a large baking dish. Add cheese and jalapenos.

5. Bake for fifteen minutes.

6. Combine scallion with sour cream in a bowl.

7. Serve the beef casserole hot with a spoonful of the sour cream mixture, green salad, and guacamole.

Keto Chicken and Roasted Veggies

Total Prep & Cooking Time: Forty-five minutes
Yields: Four servings
Nutrition Facts: Calories: 1060.3 | Protein: 65.7g |
Carbs: 8.2g| Fat: 80.3g | Fiber: 6.1g

Ingredients
For the roasted veggies:
- One pound of Brussels sprouts
- Eight ounces of cherry tomatoes
- Six ounces of mushrooms
- One tsp. of salt
- Half tsp. of black pepper (ground)
- One and a half tsp. of rosemary (dried)
- Half cup of olive oil

For the chicken:
- Four chicken breasts
- One ounce of butter
- Four ounces of herb butter (to serve)

Method:
1. Preheat your oven at two hundred degrees Celsius.

2. Arrange the veggies in a greased baking dish. Add rosemary, pepper, and salt. Drizzle olive oil from the top. Mix the veggies properly.

3. Bake the vegetables for twenty minutes.

4. Heat butter in an iron skillet. Add the chicken breasts. Season with pepper and salt. Fry for five minutes.

5. Serve the fried chicken with a dollop of herb butter on top and roasted veggies by the side.

Salmon Pie

Total Prep & Cooking Time: Fifty-five minutes
Yields: Six servings
Nutrition Facts: Calories: 1046.3 | Protein: 33.4g |
Carbs: 5.8g| Fat: 98.7g | Fiber: 7.2g

Ingredients
For the pie crust:
- Three-fourth cup of almond flour
- Four tbsps. of each
  - Sesame seeds
  - Coconut flour
- One tbsp. of ground psyllium husk powder
- One tsp. of baking powder
- One pinch of salt
- Three tbsps. of olive oil
- One large egg
- Five tbsps. of water

For the filling:
- Eight ounces of salmon (smoked)
- One cup of mayonnaise
- Three large eggs
- Two tbsps. of dill (chopped)
- Half tsp. of onion powder
- One-fourth tsp. of black pepper (ground)
- Five ounces of cream cheese
- Six ounces of cheese (shredded)

Method:

1. Preheat your oven at one hundred and seventy
   degrees Celsius.

2. Place the ingredients for the pie crust in a food
   processor. Pulse for making a firm dough.

3. Use parchment paper for lining a springform
   pan.

4. Press the prepared dough into the prepared
   pan. Bake the pie crust for fifteen minutes.

5. Combine all the listed filling ingredients in a
   large bowl. Add the filling into the crust. Bake
   for thirty minutes.

6. Let the pie sit for five minutes.

7. Serve warm.

Keto Falafel

Total Prep & Cooking Time: Forty-five minutes
Yields: Four servings
Nutrition Facts: Calories: 570.3 | Protein: 27.5g |
Carbs: 5.2g| Fat: 47.2g | Fiber: 9.6g

Ingredients

- Eight ounces of mushrooms (sliced)
- Half cup of each
  - Olive oil
  - Pumpkin seeds
  - Almonds
- Three-fourth cup of protein powder
- One-fourth cup of water
- Four tbsps. of chia seeds
- Two cloves of garlic (minced)
- Two tbsps. of parsley (chopped)
- One tsp. of each
  - Onion powder
  - Salt
  - Cumin (ground)
  - Coriander seed (ground)
- One-fourth tsp. of black pepper (ground)

Method:

1. Preheat your oven at one hundred and fifty degrees Celsius.

2. Heat a large frying pan. Add the almonds along with the pumpkin seeds. Roast for four minutes.

3. Add the almonds and pumpkin seeds into a
    food processor. Pulse until a coarse mixture
    forms.

4. Heat oil in the same pan. Add the mushrooms.
    Cook for three minutes.

5. Add cooked mushrooms along with the
    remaining ingredients in the food processor.
    Add the remaining olive oil.

6. Shape the prepared mixture into balls of four
    centimeters.

7. Arrange the falafel balls on a greased baking
    tray.

8. Bake for twenty minutes.

9. Serve the falafels warm with any side dish.

Ham Croquettes

Total Prep & Cooking Time: Twenty-five minutes
Yields: Two servings
Nutrition Facts: Calories: 1321.3 | Protein: 30.6g |
Carbs: 2.2g| Fat: 125.6g | Fiber: 0.3g

Ingredients

- Half pound of ham (cured, diced)
- Two large egg whites
- Two tbsps. of oregano (minced)
- Three tbsps. of chives (minced)
- One tbsp. of cider vinegar
- Half cup of almond flour
- One cup of coconut oil

Method:

1. Pulse ham, oregano, one egg white, chives, and oregano in a food processor.

2. Whisk cider vinegar and egg white together.

3. Take a large dish and spread the flour.

4. Make balls from the ham paste using your hands. Dip the balls in the mixture of egg white. Coat in the almond flour.

5. Heat oil a large skillet. Add the croquettes. Fry for four minutes.

6. Serve warm.

Grilled Lamb Kebabs and Anchovy Salsa Verde

Total Prep & Cooking Time: Twenty-five minutes
Yields: Four servings
Nutrition Facts: Calories: 808.3 | Protein: 15.2g |
Carbs: 6.3g| Fat: 78.2g | Fiber: 5.2g

Ingredients
For the salsa verde:
- Half cup of each
  - Mint
  - Parsley
- One ounce of anchovy (fillets)
- Two tbsps. of each
  - Pine nuts
  - Capers (drained)
- One lemon (zested)
- One-fourth clove of garlic
- Half tsp. of red pepper flakes
- One cup of olive oil
- One pinch of sea salt

For the lamb kebabs:
- Eight stems of rosemary
- Eight ounces of lamb chops (cut in cubes of one-inch)
- One eggplant (trimmed, cut in pieces of one-inch)
- Pepper and salt
- One lemon
- One-fourth cup of olive oil

Method:

1. For the salsa verde: combine parsley, mint, capers, anchovies, lemon zest, pine nuts, pepper flakes, and garlic in a food processor. While pulsing, add olive oil in a slow stream. Add salt.

2. Heat a grill pan.

3. Remove all the leaves from the rosemary stems. Leave only the top leaves. Chop the leaves.

4. Season the eggplant and lamb with pepper and salt. Sprinkle rosemary on top. Zest the lemon. Add it to the mixture of lamb and eggplant. Add olive oil. Toss for combining.

5. Thread the eggplant and lamb pieces into the rosemary stems.

6. Add the kebab skewers to the grill pan. Grill for two minutes.

7. Serve the kebabs warms with salsa verde.

Keto Salmon With Tomatoes and Pistachio-Olive Tapenade

Total Prep & Cooking Time: Thirty-five minutes
Yields: Two servings
Nutrition Facts: Calories: 840.3 | Protein: 46.7g |
Carbs: 7.6g| Fat: 66.8g | Fiber: 5.2g

Ingredients
- Two ounces of green olives (pitted)
- One and a half ounce of pistachio nuts (shelled)
- Fifteen ounces of salmon fillets
- Ten ounces of cherry tomatoes
- Half tbsp. of thyme (dried)
- One-fourth cup of each
  - Dill (chopped)
  - Olive oil
- Pepper and salt

Method:
1. Preheat your oven at one hundred and eighty degrees Celsius.

2. Chop the pistachios and olives. Combine them along with a splash of olive oil in a bowl.

3. Arrange the fillets of fish in a large baking dish. Spread the mixture of olives over the fillets.

4. Arrange the tomatoes in another baking dish. Season with thyme, pepper, and salt. Drizzle olive oil on top.

5. Bake the tomatoes and fish for fifteen minutes.

6. Serve the salmon with chopped dill on top and tomatoes by the side.

Meat Pie

Total Prep & Cooking Time: One hour and ten minutes
Yields: Six servings
Nutrition Facts: Calories: 608.3 | Protein: 35.6g | Carbs: 6.5g| Fat: 49.6g | Fiber: 6.3g

Ingredients
For the pie crust:
- Three-fourth cup of almond flour
- Four tbsps. of sesame seeds
- Five tbsps. of coconut flour
- One tbsp. of ground psyllium husk powder
- Half tsp. of baking powder
- One pinch of salt
- Three tbsps. of olive oil
- One large egg
- Five tbsps. of water

For the topping:
- Eight ounces of cottage cheese
- Seven ounces of cheese (shredded)

For the filling:
- Half yellow onion (chopped)
- One clove of garlic (chopped)
- Two tbsps. of butter
- Two pounds of beef (ground)
- One tbsp. of oregano (dried)
- Pepper and salt
- Four tbsps. of tomato paste

- Half cup of water

Method:
1. Preheat your oven at one hundred and seventy degrees Celsius.

2. Heat butter in an iron skillet. Add garlic and onion. Fry for two minutes. Add the beef. Add oregano, pepper, and salt. Fry for five minutes.

3. Add the tomato paste and water. Mix well. Simmer for twenty minutes.

4. Combine all the listed crust ingredients in a food processor.

5. Use parchment paper for lining a springform pan. Add prepared crust in the lined pan. Spread the crust all over the pan. Use your fingers for pressing the crust along the sides.

6. Use a fork for pricking the crust base.

7. Bake the crust for fifteen minutes.

8. Add the beef mixture into the crust. Spread out the filling evenly.

9. Combine cheese and cottage cheese in a bowl. Spread the mixture on top of the meat filling.

10. Bake for forty minutes.

11. Serve warm.

Skillet Pizza

Total Prep & Cooking Time: Twenty-five minutes
Yields: Two servings
Nutrition Facts: Calories: 607.6 | Protein: 34.3g |
Carbs: 4.6g| Fat: 49.9g | Fiber: 1.2g

Ingredients
- Three ounces of mozzarella cheese (shredded)
- Two ounces of sausage (cooked, crumbled)
- One ounce of pepperoni slices
- One and a half ounces of green bell pepper (sliced)
- Half tsp. of Italian seasoning
- Two tbsps. of tomato sauce

Method:
1. Heat an iron skillet over medium flame.

2. Sprinkle three-fourth of the cheese on the base of the skillet.

3. Reduce the flame. Top the cheese base with bell pepper, sausage, pepperoni, and remaining cheese. Cook for four minutes.

4. Sprinkle seasoning over the pizza.

5. Remove the skillet from heat. Let the pizza sit for five minutes.

6. Cut the pizza in slices.

7. Serve warm.

Low-Carb Lasagna

Total Prep & Cooking Time: One hour and forty minutes
Yields: Twelve servings
Nutrition Facts: Calories: 413.6 | Protein: 26.9g | Carbs: 6.8g| Fat: 29.5g | Fiber: 1.3g

Ingredients
- Two tbsps. of olive oil
- Half yellow onion (chopped)
- Two cloves of garlic (minced)
- One pound of Italian sausage
- Half pound of beef (ground)
- Twenty-four ounces of marinara sauce
- Sixteen ounces of ricotta cheese
- One large egg
- Half tsp. of salt
- One and half pound of deli chicken breast (sliced)
- Three-fourth pound of mozzarella cheese (sliced)
- Four ounces of parmesan cheese

Method:
1. Preheat your oven at two hundred and twenty degrees Celsius.

2. Heat olive in a frying pan. Add garlic and onion. Fry for three minutes.

3. Add beef and sausage. Cook for five minutes. Add the marinara sauce. Simmer for four minutes.

4. Combine egg, ricotta cheese, and salt in a bowl.

5. For assembling, add half of the meat sauce on the base of a baking dish. Follow with other layers of sliced chicken breast, mozzarella cheese, ricotta cheese mixture, and parmesan cheese.

6. Repeat for the remaining ingredients. The top layer will be a layer of parmesan and mozzarella.

7. Cover the dish with aluminum foil. Bake for twenty-five minutes.

8. Remove the foil. Bake for twenty minutes.

9. Let the lasagna sit for fifteen minutes.

10. Serve warm.

Keto Pasta and Blue Cheese Sauce

Total Prep & Cooking Time: Thirty-five minutes
Yields: Four servings
Nutrition Facts: Calories: 940.7 | Protein: 35.1g |
Carbs: 8.6g| Fat: 81.4g | Fiber: 12.1g

Ingredients
For the blue cheese sauce:
- Seven ounces of each
  - Cream cheese
  - Blue cheese
- Two ounces of butter
- Two tsps. of pepper

For serving:
- Four tbsps. of pine nuts (roasted)
- Two ounces of parmesan cheese (grated)

For the pasta:
- Eight large eggs
- Ten ounces of cream cheese
- One tsp. of salt
- Six tbsps. of ground psyllium husk powder

Method:
1. Preheat your oven at one hundred and fifty degrees Celsius.

2. Mix cream cheese, eggs, and salt. Add the psyllium husk powder. Let the batter sit for two minutes.

3. Use parchment paper for lining a baking tray.
   Use a spatula for spreading the batter on the
   tray. Top with another parchment paper.
   Flatten the batter using a rolling pin. Bake for
   twelve minutes.

4. Use a pizza slicer for cutting the pasta into very
   thin strips.

5. Combine blue cheese along with cream cheese
   in a saucepan. Stir for five minutes.

6. Add the butter. Warm the sauce for two
   minutes. Add the pepper.

7. Serve the pasta with blue cheese sauce on top.
   Garnish with parmesan cheese and pine nuts.

BBQ Chicken Meatza

Total Prep & Cooking Time: Forty minutes
Yields: Four servings
Nutrition Facts: Calories: 746.3 | Protein: 58.6g |
Carbs: 4.9g| Fat: 53.4g | Fiber: 1.6g

Ingredients
For the crust:
- One pound of chicken (ground)
- Half tsp. of salt
- Ten ounces of parmesan cheese (grated)

For the BBQ sauce:
- Half cup of tomato sauce
- One tsp. of cider vinegar
- One-fourth tsp. of each
  - Garlic powder
  - Onion powder
- Half tsp. of liquid smoke
- One pinch of salt

For the toppings:
- Five ounces of cheddar cheese (shredded)
- Half red onion (sliced)
- Six ounces of bacon

Method:
1. Preheat your oven at two hundred degrees Celsius.

2. Combine parmesan cheese, ground chicken, and salt.

3. Use parchment paper for lining a baking sheet. Press the mixture of crust on the baking sheet. Bake for fifteen minutes.

4. For the BBQ sauce, combine vinegar, liquid smoke, tomato sauce, garlic powder, onion powder, and salt in a bowl.

5. Spread the BBQ sauce over the pizza. Top with red onion and cheddar cheese. Bake for seven minutes.

6. Cook the bacon in an iron skillet for three minutes.

7. Let the pizza sit for two minutes. Serve with crispy bacon on top.

Chicken Alfredo Pasta

Total Prep & Cooking Time: One hour and ten minutes
Yields: Four servings
Nutrition Facts: Calories: 1214.3 | Protein: 75.3g | Carbs: 8.8g| Fat: 107.2g | Fiber: 21.1g

Ingredients
For the pasta:
- Four large eggs
- Six egg yolks
- Three-fourth cup of water
- Two tbsps. of olive oil
- Half cup of ground psyllium husk powder
- Four tbsps. of coconut flour
- Three tsps. of herbal salt

For the sauce:
- Two pounds of chicken breast
- Ten ounces of bacon (fried)
- One and a half cup of whipping cream
- Three-fourth cup of milk (whole)
- Three ounces of parmesan cheese
- Four cloves of garlic (minced)
- Four tbsps. of green pesto
- Pepper and salt
- Eight mushrooms (sliced)
- One red bell pepper (sliced)
- Butter (to fry)

Method:

1. Preheat your oven at one hundred and fifty
    degrees Celsius.

2. Combine olive oil, eggs, and other liquids in a
    bowl. Add the dry ingredients into the egg
    batter. Let the batter sit for eight minutes.

3. Use parchment paper for lining a baking sheet.
    Add the batter. Top with another parchment
    paper. Use a rolling pin for flattening the
    batter.

4. Remove the top parchment paper. Bake for ten
    minutes. Use a sharp knife for cutting into
    strips.

5. Preheat your oven at two hundred degrees
    Celsius.

6. Split the chicken breast lengthwise. Add pepper
    and salt.

7. Heat butter in an iron skillet. Add the chicken.
    Fry for ten minutes.

8. Remove the chicken.

9. In the same skillet, fry the bacon. Add
    parmesan cheese, milk, and cream. Boil the
    mixture. Add pesto, chopped garlic, pepper,
    and salt.

10. Fry mushrooms and peppers in an iron skillet
    with butter. Add pepper and salt. Add the
    pasta. Mix well.

11. Pour the sauce over the pasta. Mix well.
    Simmer for two minutes.

12. Serve the pasta with cooked chicken on top.
    Garnish with parmesan cheese.

Cauliflower Alfredo

Total Prep & Cooking Time: Forty-five minutes
Yields: Four servings
Nutrition Facts: Calories: 1002.3 | Protein: 56.6g |
Carbs: 7.9g| Fat: 80.3g | Fiber: 4.3g

Ingredients

- Five ounces of bacon (diced)
- Two pounds of chicken breast
- Two ounces of butter
- Four cloves of garlic (minced)
- Seven ounces of baby spinach
- Two cups of whipping cream
- Four ounces of parmesan cheese (grated)
- Pepper and salt
- Two and a half pounds of cauliflower

Method:

1. Start by frying the bacon in an iron skillet. Keep aside.

2. Slice the chicken breast into strips.

3. Heat butter in the same skillet. Add bacon fat and garlic. Fry the chicken strips for five minutes.

4. Sauté the spinach in a pan. Cook until the leaves wilt.

5. Add the cream in the pan. Boil for two minutes. Add bacon, parmesan cheese, and chicken. Add pepper and salt.

6. Simmer for five minutes.

7. Chop the cauliflower into small florets. Parboil the florets in salted water for three minutes. Drain the water.

8. Add the cauliflower in the mixture of chicken.

9. Mix well. Serve hot.

Chicken Wings With Creamed Broccoli

Total Prep & Cooking Time: Fifty-five minutes
Yields: Four servings
Nutrition Facts: Calories: 1120.3 | Protein: 64.9g |
Carbs: 8.6g| Fat: 98.3g | Fiber: 5.6g

Ingredients
For the chicken wings:
- Half orange (juiced, zested)
- One-fourth cup of olive oil
- Two tsps. of ginger (ground)
- One tsp. of salt
- One-fourth tsp. of cayenne pepper
- Three pounds of chicken wings

For the broccoli:
- Two pounds of broccoli
- One cup of mayonnaise
- One-fourth cup of dill (chopped)
- Pepper and salt

Method:
1. Preheat your oven at two hundred degrees Celsius.

2. Combine orange zest, juice, spices, and oil in a bowl. Add the chicken. Mix well. Marinate for five minutes.

3. Arrange the wings in a greased baking tray. Bake for forty minutes.

4. Chop the broccoli into small florets. Parboil the florets in salted water for four minutes. Drain the water.

5. Add the broccoli florets in a bowl along with the remaining ingredients. Mix well.

6. Serve the chicken wings with creamy broccoli by the side.

Chicken Provencale

Total Prep & Cooking Time: One hour and fifteen minutes
Yields: Four servings
Nutrition Facts: Calories: 908.3 | Protein: 44.3g | Carbs: 5.3g| Fat: 80.3g | Fiber: 3.3g

Ingredients
- Two pounds of chicken drumsticks
- Eight ounces of tomatoes
- Three ounces of black olives (pitted)
- One-fourth cup of olive oil
- Five cloves of garlic (sliced)
- One tbsp. of oregano (dried)
- Pepper and salt

For serving:
- Seven ounces of lettuce
- One cup of mayonnaise
- One-fourth lemon (zested)
- One tsp. of paprika powder
- Pepper and salt

Method:
1. Preheat your oven at two hundred degrees Celsius. Arrange the chicken in a baking dish with the skin side up. Add olives, garlic, tomatoes around the meat.

2. Drizzle some olive oil over the chicken. Add pepper, salt, and oregano.

3. Roast in the oven for one hour.

4. Combine lettuce, mayo, paprika, lemon zest, pepper, and salt in a bowl. Mix well.

5. Serve the chicken with lettuce mix by the side.

Tuna Cheese Melt

Total Prep & Cooking Time: Fifty-five minutes
Yields: Four servings
Nutrition Facts: Calories: 912.3 | Protein: 38.6g |
Carbs: 5.6g| Fat: 80.1g | Fiber: 3.3g

Ingredients
For the bread:
- Three large eggs
- Five ounces of cream cheese
- One pinch of salt
- Half tbsp. of ground psyllium husk powder
- Half tsp. of baking powder

For the tuna mix:
- One cup of mayonnaise
- Four stalks of celery
- Two ounces of dill pickles (chopped)
- Eight ounces of tuna in olive oil
- One clove of garlic (minced)
- One tsp. of lemon juice
- Pepper and salt

For the topping:
- Ten ounces of cheese (shredded)
- One-fourth tsp. of cayenne pepper

For serving:

- Olive oil
- Five ounces of leafy greens

Method:

1. For the bread, preheat your oven at one hundred and fifty degrees Celsius.

2. Separate the egg whites and yolks.

3. Add salt in the egg whites. Keep whipping until stiff mixture forms.

4. Combine cream cheese and egg yolks. Add baking powder and psyllium husk powder.

5. Fold the mixture of egg whites into the mixture of egg yolks. Divide the mixture into two portions and add them in a lined baking sheet.

6. Bake for twenty minutes.

7. For the assembly, preheat your oven at one hundred seventy degrees Celsius.

8. Combine all the listed ingredients for the tuna mix in a large bowl.

9. Cut the bread slices in half. Top each half with the mixture of tuna. Add cheese on top.

10. Sprinkle paprika powder from the top.

11. Bake for fifteen minutes.

12. Serve the tuna sandwich with olive oil and leafy greens.

Sesame Salmon and Thai Curry Cabbage

Total Prep & Cooking Time: Forty minutes
Yields: Four servings
Nutrition Facts: Calories: 1051.6 | Protein: 37.9g |
Carbs: 8.2g| Fat: 95.4g | Fiber: 7.6g

Ingredients
For the lime mayonnaise:
- One cup of mayonnaise
- Half lime (juiced, zested)

For the Thai curry cabbage:
- Two tbsps. of coconut oil
- Two pounds of green cabbage (shredded)
- One tbsp. of red curry paste
- Half tbsp. of sesame oil
- Pepper and salt

For the salmon:
- Two pounds of salmon pieces
- Two tbsps. of sesame seeds
- Three ounces of butter
- One lime
- Pepper and salt

Method:
1. Combine the listed ingredients for the lime mayo in a bowl. Mix well. Leave the lime mayo in the refrigerator.

2. Heat oil in a steel wok. Add the curry paste along with the cabbage. Sauté for four minutes. Add pepper and salt. Add the sesame oil. Toss for two minutes.

3. Add pepper and salt to the salmon. Dip the pieces of fish in sesame seeds for coating.

4. Heat butter in an iron skillet. Fry the salmon pieces for four minutes.

5. Serve the salmon with Thai curry cabbage and lime mayo by the side.

Grilled White Fish and Zucchini With Kale Pesto

Total Prep & Cooking Time: Twenty-five minutes
Yields: Four servings
Nutrition Facts: Calories: 775.3 | Protein: 37.2g |
Carbs: 6.9g| Fat: 68.3g | Fiber: 3.2g

Ingredients
For the kale pesto:
- Three ounces of kale
- Three tbsps. of lemon juice
- Two ounces of walnuts
- One clove of garlic
- Half tsp. of salt
- One-fourth tsp. of black pepper (ground)
- Three-fourth cup of olive oil

For the fish and zucchini:
- Two zucchinis
- One tbsp. of lemon juice
- Half tsp. of salt
- Two tbsps. of olive oil
- Two pounds of white fish
- One-fourth tsp. of black pepper (ground)

Method:
1. Roughly chop the kale. Add kale, lemon juice, walnuts, and garlic in a high power blender. Blend until smooth. Add pepper and salt. Add olive oil. Blend again for one minute.

2. Cut thin strips from the zucchini. Toss zucchini slices with pepper, salt, olive oil, and lemon juice.

3. Season the fish pieces with salt. Brush the pieces of fish with oil.

4. Heat a grill pan. Add the fish. Grill for three minutes on all sides.

5. Serve the fish with zucchini and kale pesto by the side.

Chapter 8: Easy Keto Snack Recipes

No matter which diet you follow, having mid-meal cravings is very natural. So, I have included some tasty yet easy snack recipes in this chapter that you can include in your keto diet plan.

Tuscan Truffles

Total Prep & Cooking Time: Twenty-five minutes
Yields: Six servings
Nutrition Facts: Calories: 82.3 | Protein: 3.3g | Carbs: 1.6g| Fat: 7.3g | Fiber: 0.6g

Ingredients

- Two logs of goat cheese
- Eight ounces of mascarpone cheese
- Six tbsps. of parmesan cheese (grated)
- Three cloves of garlic (minced)
- Two tsps. of olive oil
- One tsp. of white balsamic vinegar
- Three-fourth tsp. of lemon zest (grated)
- Six and a half tbsp. of prosciutto (chopped)
- Five tbsps. of dried figs (chopped)
- Three tbsps. of parsley (minced)
- One-fourth tsp. of pepper
- One cup of pine nuts (chopped)

Method:

1. Mix the first eleven listed ingredients in a large
    bowl.

2. Shape the mixture into thirty-six small balls.

3. Roll the balls in chopped pine nuts.

4. Refrigerate for twenty minutes.

Caprese Salad Kabobs

Total Prep & Cooking Time: Ten minutes
Yields: Four servings
Nutrition Facts: Calories: 45.4 | Protein: 2.3g | Carbs: 1.6g| Fat: 5.1g | Fiber: 1.2g

Ingredients
- Twenty-four grape tomatoes
- Twelve small bits of mozzarella cheese balls
- Twenty-four basil leaves.
- Two tbsps. of olive oil
- Two tsps. of balsamic vinegar

Method:
1. Combine vinegar along with olive oil in a small bowl.

2. Thread two tomatoes, two leaves of basil, and one ball of cheese alternately on each skewer.

3. Drizzle the mixture of olive oil over the skewers.

4. Serve immediately.

Roasted Cauliflower and Tahini Yogurt Sauce

Total Prep & Cooking Time: Fifty-five minutes
Yields: Four servings
Nutrition Facts: Calories: 179.6 | Protein: 7.6g |
Carbs: 5.1g| Fat: 15.4g | Fiber: 2.2g

Ingredients

- One-fourth cup of parmesan cheese (grated)
- Three tbsps. of olive oil
- Two cloves of garlic (minced)
- One-fourth tsp. of salt
- One-third tsp. of pepper
- One cauliflower (cut in four wedges)

For the sauce:
- Half cup of Greek yogurt
- One tbsp. of lemon juice
- Half tbsp. of tahini
- One-fourth tsp. of salt
- One pinch of paprika
- Parsley (minced)

Method:

1. Preheat your oven at one hundred and fifty degrees Celsius.

2. Mix the first five ingredients.

3. Rub the mixture over the wedges of cauliflower.

4. Grease a baking tray with cooking spray.

5. Arrange the wedges of cauliflower on the baking tray. Roast for forty minutes.

6. For the sauce, combine lemon juice, yogurt, seasonings, and tahini in a bowl.

7. Serve the cauliflower wedges and drizzle tahini sauce on top. Garnish with parsley.

Zucchini Crusted Pizza

Total Prep & Cooking Time: Forty-five minutes
Yields: Six servings
Nutrition Facts: Calories: 226.3 | Protein: 13.6g |
Carbs: 8.6g| Fat: 11.6g | Fiber: 1.6g

Ingredients
- Two large eggs (beaten)
- Two cups of zucchini (shredded, squeezed)
- Half cup of mozzarella cheese (shredded)
- One-third cup of parmesan cheese (grated)
- One-fourth cup of flour
- One tbsp. of olive oil
- One and a half tbsp. of basil (minced)
- One tsp. of thyme (minced)

For the toppings:
- Twelve ounces of sweet red pepper (roasted, julienned)
- One cup of mozzarella cheese (shredded)
- Half cup of turkey pepperoni (sliced)

Method:
1. Preheat your oven at two hundred degrees Celsius.

2. Combine the first eight listed ingredients in a bowl.

3. Transfer the mixture to a greased pizza pan. Spread the mixture and evenly press it to the base.

4. Bake for sixteen minutes.

5. Add the toppings on the pizza. Bake for twelve
    minutes.

6.   Slice the pizza using a pizza cutter.

7. Serve hot.

<u>Stuffed Basil- Asiago Mushrooms</u>

Total Prep & Cooking Time: Thirty-five minutes
Yields: Four servings
Nutrition Facts: Calories: 36.6 | Protein: 2.3g | Carbs: 1.5g| Fat: 3.3g | Fiber: 0.3g

Ingredients

- Twenty-four Portobello mushrooms (remove the stems)
- Half cup of mayonnaise
- Three-fourth cup of Asiago cheese(shredded)
- One-third cup of basil leaves (remove the stems)
- One-fourth tsp. of white pepper
- Twelve cherry tomatoes (halved)

Method:

1. Preheat your oven at one hundred and fifty degrees Celsius.

2. Grease a baking dish with cooking spray.

3. Arrange the mushroom caps in the dish. Bake the mushrooms for ten minutes.

4. Combine Asiago cheese, mayonnaise, pepper, and basil in a food processor. Mix well.

5. Fill the mushroom caps with the cheese and basil mixture. Top each mushroom cap with half a tomato.

6. Bake for ten minutes.

7. Serve warm.

Cheese and Zucchini Roulades

Total Prep & Cooking Time: Twenty-five minutes
Yields: Six servings
Nutrition Facts: Calories: 29.4 | Protein: 3.5g | Carbs: 1.2g| Fat: 1.6g | Fiber: 0.2g

Ingredients

- One cup of ricotta cheese
- One-fourth cup of parmesan cheese (grated)
- Two tbsps. of basil (minced)
- One tbsp. of capers
- One and a half tbsp. of Greek olives (chopped)
- One tsp. of lemon zest (grated)
- Two tbsps. of lemon juice
- One-eighth tsp. of pepper
- One-fourth tsp. of salt
- Four zucchinis

Method:

1. Combine the first nine listed ingredients in a bowl.

2. Slice the zucchinis into twenty-four slices lengthwise.

3. Grease a grill rack with cooking spray.

4. Cook the slices of zucchini for three minutes.

5. Add one tbsp. of the ricotta cheese mixture on one end of the zucchini slices.

6. Roll up the slices. Secure using toothpicks.

7. Serve immediately.

Chicken Nuggets With Sweet Potato Crusting

Total Prep & Cooking Time: Thirty minutes
Yields: Four servings
Nutrition Facts: Calories: 305.6 | Protein: 26.6g |
Carbs: 8.6g| Fat: 18.9g | Fiber: 1.6g

Ingredients

- One cup of sweet potato chips
- One-fourth cup of flour
- One tsp. of salt
- Half tsp. of ground pepper (ground)
- One-fourth tsp. of baking powder
- One tbsp. of cornstarch
- One pound of chicken tenderloins (cut in pieces of half-inch)
- Oil (to fry)

Method:

1. Heat the oil in a large skillet.

2. Add flour, chips, salt, baking powder, and pepper in a food processor. Pulse the ingredients for making a ground mixture.

3. Toss the chicken pieces in cornstarch. Shake off excess cornstarch. Toss in the chip mixture. Press the chicken pieces gently for coating.

4. Fry the chicken nuggets for three minutes.

5. Serve hot.

Artichoke and Spinach Stuffed Mushrooms

Total Prep & Cooking Time: Forty minutes
Yields: Six servings
Nutrition Facts: Calories: 52.2 | Protein: 2.6g | Carbs: 1.5g| Fat: 5.6g | Fiber: 0.2g

Ingredients
- Three ounces of cream cheese
- Half cup of mayonnaise
- One cup of sour cream
- Three-fourth tsp. of garlic salt
- One can of artichoke hearts (chopped)
- Ten ounces of spinach (chopped)
- One-third cup of mozzarella cheese (shredded)
- Three tbsps. of parmesan cheese (shredded)
- Thirty large mushrooms (remove the stems)

Method:
1. Preheat your oven at two hundred degrees Celsius.

2. Combine the first four listed ingredients in a bowl.

3. Add spinach, artichoke, three tbsps. of parmesan cheese, and mozzarella cheese.

4. Arrange the mushrooms on a large aluminum foil-lined baking tray.

5. Add one tbsp. of the filling into the mushroom
    caps. Sprinkle remaining parmesan cheese
    from the top.

6. Bake for twenty minutes.

Cobb Salad Sausage Lettuce Wraps

Total Prep & Cooking Time: Twenty-five minutes
Yields: Six servings
Nutrition Facts: Calories: 430.6 | Protein: 16.5g |
Carbs: 5.8g| Fat: 39.6g | Fiber: 3.5g

Ingredients
- Three-fourth cup of ranch salad dressing
- One-third cup of blue cheese (crumbled)
- One-fourth cup of watercress (chopped)
- One pound of pork sausage
- Two tbsps. of chives (minced)
- Six leaves of iceberg lettuce
- One avocado (peeled, diced)
- Four boiled eggs (chopped)
- One tomato (chopped)

Method:
1. Combine blue cheese, dressing, and watercress in a bowl.

2. Heat some oil in an iron skillet. Add the sausage. Cook for seven minutes and crumble. Add the chives.

3. Spoon the sausage mixture into the leaves of lettuce. Top the sausage mixture with eggs, tomato, and avocado. Drizzle the mixture of dressing on top.

4. Serve immediately.

Mushroom and Asparagus Frittata

Total Prep & Cooking Time: Forty-five minutes
Yields: Eight servings
Nutrition Facts: Calories: 132.3 | Protein: 9.3g |
Carbs: 5.1g| Fat: 8.2g | Fiber: 1.6g

Ingredients

- Eight large eggs
- Half cup of ricotta cheese
- Two tbsps. of lemon juice
- Half tsp. of salt
- One-fourth tsp. of pepper
- One tbsp. of olive oil
- Eight ounces of asparagus spears
- One onion (sliced)
- One-third cup of sweet green pepper
- Three-fourth cup of Portobello mushrooms (sliced)

Method:

1. Preheat your oven at one hundred and fifty degrees Celsius.

2. Combine ricotta cheese, eggs, pepper, lemon juice, and salt in a bowl.

3. Heat oil in an iron skillet. Add onion, asparagus, mushrooms, and red pepper. Cook for eight minutes. Remove the asparagus from the skillet.

4. Cut the spears of asparagus into pieces of two-inch. Return the spears to the skillet.

5. Add the mixture of eggs.

6. Bake in the oven for twenty minutes.

7. Let the frittata sit for five minutes.

8. Cut the frittata into wedges. Serve warm.

Sausage Balls

Total Prep & Cooking Time: Forty-five minutes
Yields: Six servings
Nutrition Facts: Calories: 102.3 | Protein: 5.9g |
Carbs: 0.7g| Fat: 9.6g | Fiber: 0.2g

Ingredients

- One pound of spicy pork sausage (ground)
- Eight ounces of cream cheese
- Half cup of cheddar cheese (shredded)
- One-third cup of parmesan cheese (shredded)
- One tbsp. of Dijon mustard
- Half tsp. of garlic powder
- One-fourth tsp. of salt

Method:

1. Preheat your oven at one hundred and seventy degrees Celsius.

2. Use parchment paper for lining a baking sheet.

3. Combine cream cheese, sausage, parmesan cheese, cheddar cheese, garlic powder, mustard, and salt in a mixing bowl. Mix well.

4. Take one tbsp. of the mixture. Roll it into a ball. Repeat for the remaining mixture.

5. Arrange the prepared balls on the lined baking tray.

6. Bake for thirty minutes.

7. Serve hot.

Ranch Cauliflower Crackers

Total Prep & Cooking Time: One hour and ten minutes
Yields: Six servings
Nutrition Facts: Calories: 29.6 | Protein: 2.6g | Carbs: 1.1g| Fat: 2.6g | Fiber: 0.6g

Ingredients

- Twelve ounces of cauliflower rice
- Cheesecloth
- One large egg
- One tbsp. of ranch salad dressing mix (dry)
- One-eighth tsp. of cayenne pepper
- One cup of parmesan cheese (shredded)

Method:

1. Add the cauliflower rice in a large bowl. Microwave for four minutes covered.

2. Transfer the cauliflower rice to a strainer lined with cheesecloth. Squeeze out excess moisture.

3. Preheat oven at two hundred degrees Celsius. Use parchment paper for lining a baking tray.

4. Combine egg, cauliflower rice, ranch mix, and pepper in a bowl. Add the cheese. Mix well.

5. Take two tbsps. of the mixture and add them to the baking tray. Flatten with your hands. The thinner you can make the mixture, the crispier will be the crackers.

6. Bake for ten minutes. Flip the crackers. Bake
    for ten minutes.

7. Serve warm.

Pork Belly Cracklins

Total Prep & Cooking Time: One hour and thirty-five minutes
Yields: Six servings
Nutrition Facts: Calories: 210.3 | Protein: 16.5g |
Carbs: 1.5g| Fat: 16.6g | Fiber: 0.3g

Ingredients
- Three pounds of pork belly (with skin)
- Two cups of water
- Four tbsps. of Cajun seasoning

Method:
1. Keep the pork belly in the refrigerator for forty minutes.

2. Cut the pork into cubes of three-fourth inch.

3. Fill a cast-iron pot with one-fourth portion of water. Add one tsp. of Cajun seasoning. Boil the water.

4. Add the cubes of pork belly.

5. Cook for twenty minutes.

6. Cover the pot once fat begins to pop and sizzle. Cook for fifteen minutes.

7. Drain the pork cracklins.

8. Sprinkle remaining seasoning from the top.

9. Serve immediately.

Lemon Fat Bombs

Total Prep & Cooking Time: Fifty minutes
Yields: Four servings
Nutrition Facts: Calories: 69.9 | Protein: 0.5g | Carbs: 2.6g| Fat: 7.9g | Fiber: 1.1g

Ingredients
- One cup of shredded coconut (dry)
- One-fourth cup of coconut oil
- Three tbsps. of erythritol sweetener (powdered)
- Two tbsps. of lemon zest
- One pinch of salt

Method:
1. Add the coconut in a high power blender. Blend until creamy for fifteen minutes.

2. Add sweetener, coconut oil, salt, and lemon zest. Blend for two minutes.

3. Fill small muffin cups with the coconut mixture.

4. Chill in the refrigerator for thirty minutes.

Peanut Butter Granola

Total Prep & Cooking Time: Forty minutes
Yields: Twelve servings
Nutrition Facts: Calories: 335.9 | Protein: 10.6g |
Carbs: 7.8g| Fat: 31.2g | Fiber: 5.2g

Ingredients
- Two cups of each
  - Almonds
  - Pecans
- One cup of shredded coconut
- One-fourth cup of each
  - Sunflower seeds
  - Water
  - Butter
- One-third cup of each
  - Sweetener
  - Vanilla protein powder
  - Peanut butter

Method:
1. Preheat your oven at one hundred and fifty degrees Celsius.

2. Use parchment paper for lining a large baking tray.

3. Add pecans and almonds in a blender. Process for two minutes.

4. Combine processed mixture with sweetener, coconut, vanilla protein powder, and sunflower seeds.

5. Melt butter along with peanut butter in a bowl.

6. Add melted butter mixture over the mixture of nuts. Mix well.

7. Spread the nut mixture on the baking tray evenly.

8. Bake for thirty minutes.

Hot Chocolate

Total Prep & Cooking Time: Ten minutes
Yields: One serving
Nutrition Facts: Calories: 211.6 | Protein: 15.6g |
Carbs: 3.6g| Fat: 17.6g | Fiber: 2.6g

Ingredients

- Half cup of almond milk
- Two tbsps. of whipping cream
- One tbsp. of cocoa powder
- One and a half tbsp. of caramel collagen (salted)
- Sweetener
- Whipped cream (to serve)
- Caramel sauce (to serve)

Method:

1. Combine whipping cream and almond milk in a saucepan.

2. Add collagen and cocoa powder in a blender. Add the milk mixture. Keep blending until frothy. Adjust the sweetness.

3. Pour the hot chocolate in serving cup.

4. Top with whipped cream and caramel sauce.

Choco Chip Cookies

Total Prep & Cooking Time: Thirty minutes
Yields: Five servings
Nutrition Facts: Calories: 239.3 | Protein: 5.6g |
Carbs: 7.1g| Fat: 23.2g | Fiber: 3.6g

Ingredients
- Two cups of almond flour
- Three-fourth cup of unsweetened shredded coconut
- One tsp. of baking powder
- Half tsp. of each
  - Salt
  - Vanilla extract
- Half cup of butter
- One-third cup of sweetener
- Two tsps. of molasses
- One large egg
- One-fourth cup of chocolate chips

Method:
1. Preheat your oven at one hundred and fifty degrees Celsius.

2. Use parchment paper for lining a baking tray.

3. Whisk baking powder, coconut, almond flour, and salt.

4. Mix butter, molasses, along with sweetener. Add egg and vanilla extract. Mix well.

5. Add the mixture of flour. Combine for making a firm dough.

6. Add the chocolate chips.

7. Shape the prepared dough into balls of two-inch. Place them on the baking tray. Press the balls for flattening them.

8. Bake for fifteen minutes.

9. Let the cookies sit for five minutes.

Jalapeno Cheddar Meatballs

Total Prep & Cooking Time: Fifty minutes
Yields: Eight servings
Nutrition Facts: Calories: 366.5 | Protein: 34.3g |
Carbs: 1.3g| Fat: 25.4g | Fiber: 0.4g

Ingredients
- Two pounds of beef (ground)
- Six ounces of cheddar cheese (grated)
- Half cup of pork rind (crumbs)
- One large egg
- One jalapeno (diced)
- Two tbsps. of cilantro (chopped)
- One tsp. of chili powder
- One-fourth tsp. of garlic powder
- One and a half tsp. of salt
- One-third tsp. of each
    - Pepper
    - Cumin

Method:
1. Preheat your oven at one hundred and fifty degrees Celsius. Use parchment paper for lining a baking tray.

2. Add all the listed ingredients in a high power blender. Process until combined properly.

3. Roll two-inch balls from the mixture using your hands. Place the balls on the baking tray.

4. Bake for twenty minutes.

5. Serve hot.

Pepperoni Pizza Bites

Total Prep & Cooking Time: Twenty minutes
Yields: Six servings
Nutrition Facts: Calories: 82.1 | Protein: 5.2g | Carbs:
1.1g| Fat: 5.9g | Fiber: 0.3g

Ingredients
- Twenty-four pepperoni slices
- Twenty-four basil leaves
- One jar of pizza sauce
- Twenty-four balls of mozzarella cheese
- Black olives (sliced)

Method:
1. Preheat your oven at two hundred degrees
   Celsius.

2. Use a sharp knife for snipping four cuts of half-
   inch around the pepperoni slice edges.

3. Press the slices into muffin cups of a muffin tin.
   Bake for six minutes.

4. Add one basil leaf at the base of each cup. Top
   with half tsp. of pizza sauce, olive slice, and
   mozzarella ball.

5. Bake for three minutes. Let the pizza cups sit
   for two minutes.

6. Serve warm.

Cream Cheese and Bacon Pinwheels

Total Prep & Cooking Time: Twenty minutes
Yields: Ten servings
Nutrition Facts: Calories: 145.3 | Protein: 7.6g |
Carbs: 2.1g| Fat: 13.2g | Fiber: 1.2g

Ingredients

- Eight ham slices (sliced)
- Five slices of bacon (cooked)
- Four ounces of cream cheese (softened)
- Two tsps. of ranch seasoning
- One-fourth cup of olives (chopped)

Method:

1. Arrange the slices of ham on a working surface. Overlap the slices in rows of four by two.

2. Spread the softened cream cheese evenly all over the ham.

3. Sprinkle seasoning on the layer of cream cheese. Arrange the olives on the cream cheese.

4. Add the strips of bacon on the cream cheese layer.

5. Roll the pinwheels carefully. Roll as tightly as you can.

6. Carefully hold the roll. Cut into pieces of half-inch.

7. Serve immediately.

<u>*Sausage Rolls*</u>

Total Prep & Cooking Time: Fifty minutes
Yields: Six servings
Nutrition Facts: Calories: 477.6 | Protein: 27.2g |
Carbs: 4.5g| Fat: 40.3g | Fiber: 1.6g

Ingredients
For the sausage rolls:
- Five hundred grams of sausage
- Onion flakes (to garnish)

For the fat head pastry:
- One hundred and seventy grams of mozzarella cheese (grated)
- Half cup of almond flour
- Two tbsps. of cream cheese
- One large egg
- One pinch of salt
- One tsp. of onion flakes

Method:
1. Arrange the sausages on a baking tray. Bake for ten minutes at one hundred and eighty degrees Celsius.

2. Combine almond flour along with cheese in a bowl. Mix the cream cheese. Microwave the prepared mixture on high settings for one minute.

3. Add salt, egg, and onion flakes. Combine properly.

4. Place the pastry dough between two parchment paper sheets. Flatten the dough with the help of a rolling pin.

5. Cut the pastry dough into strips that are wide enough for rolling the sausages.

6. Add the sausages in the strips and roll.

7. Cut each roll into four to five pieces for making mini sausage rolls.

8. Sprinkle onion flakes on top.

9. Bake for fifteen minutes at two hundred degrees Celsius.

10. Serve hot.

Dill Garlic Baked Cucumber Chips

Total Prep & Cooking Time: Three hours and fifteen minutes
Yields: Eight servings
Nutrition Facts: Calories: 16.3 | Protein: 0.9g | Carbs: 2.2g| Fat: 0.2g | Fiber: 0.6g

Ingredients
- Two cucumbers
- One tbsp. of dill (dried)
- One tsp. of each
  - Garlic powder
  - Onion powder
- One-fourth tbsp. of apple cider vinegar
- Salt

Method:
1. Slice the cucumbers into thin slices of one-eighth inch.

2. Line the slices of cucumber on a paper towel. Add another towel over the cucumber slices. Gently press for removing excess moisture.

3. Add the cucumber slices in a bowl.

4. Preheat your oven at two hundred degrees Celsius.

5. Combine onion powder, dill, apple cider vinegar, and garlic powder in a small bowl.

6. Add the mixture of herbs over the cucumber slices. Toss well for combining.

7. Arrange the tossed cucumber slices on a baking tray. Sprinkle salt on top.

8. Bake the cucumber slices of three hours.

9. Let the cucumber chips sit in the oven for three minutes.

10. Serve warm.

Mozzarella Sticks

Total Prep & Cooking Time: Fifty minutes
Yields: Four servings
Nutrition Facts: Calories: 388.6 | Protein: 37.6g |
Carbs: 2.6g| Fat: 29.6g | Fiber: 1.2g

Ingredients
- Six mozzarella string cheese sticks (halved)
- Two tbsps. of parmesan cheese (grated)
- One tbsp. of coconut flour
- One tsp. of baking powder
- Half tsp. of garlic powder
- One and a half tsp. of Italian seasoning
- One large egg
- Pepper and salt

Method:
1. Combine egg, pepper, and salt in a bowl.

2. Mix all the dry listed ingredients.

3. Dip the sticks of cheese into the beaten egg. Roll the sticks in the parmesan cheese mixture for coating. Repeat again for double coating.

4. Chill the coated mozzarella sticks in the refrigerator for thirty minutes.

5. Heat oil in a large pan.

6. Fry the cheese sticks for one minute.

7. Serve warm.

Soft Pretzel

Total Prep & Cooking Time: Thirty minutes
Yields: Three servings
Nutrition Facts: Calories: 456.3 | Protein: 28.7g |
Carbs: 7.6g| Fat: 36.6g | Fiber: 4.6g

Ingredients
- Two cups of almond flour
- One tbsp. of baking powder
- One tsp. of garlic powder
- One and a half tsp. of onion powder
- Three large eggs
- Three cups of mozzarella cheese (shredded)
- Five tbsps. of cream cheese
- Sea salt

Method:
1. Preheat your oven at two hundred degrees Celsius.

2. Use parchment paper for lining a baking tray.

3. Combine baking powder, almond flour, onion powder, and garlic powder in a bowl. Add two eggs in the mixture. Mix well.

4. Combine cream cheese along with mozzarella cheese in a bowl. Microwave for two minutes.

5. Add the cheese mixture to the dough. Mix well.

6. Beat one egg in a small bowl.

7. Divide prepared dough into six portions. Roll each of them into thin sticks. Fold the sticks for shaping like pretzels.

8. Use egg wash for brushing the top portion of the pretzels.

9. Sprinkle salt on top.

10. Bake for fifteen minutes.

Dill Pickle Almonds

Total Prep & Cooking Time: Thirty minutes
Yields: Six servings
Nutrition Facts: Calories: 208.3 | Protein: 8.6g |
Carbs: 5.3g| Fat: 18.2g | Fiber: 3.6g

Ingredients
- One large egg white
- Three cups of almonds
- Two tsps. of citric acid
- Two and a half tsp. of salt
- Three tsps. of dill (dried)
- Three-fourth tsp. of garlic powder
- Half tsp. of pepper
- One-fourth tsp. of coriander

Method:
1. Preheat your oven at one hundred and fifty degrees Celsius.

2. Use parchment paper for lining a baking tray.

3. Whisk the egg white in a bowl. Keep whisking until frothy. Add the almonds. Mix well.

4. Add salt, citric acid, pepper, garlic powder, coriander, and dill. Toss for combining.

5. Bake the coated almonds for twelve minutes.

6. Let the almonds sit for five minutes in the oven.

7. Serve warm.

<u>Strawberry Cheesecake Popsicle</u>

Total Prep & Cooking Time: Four hours and fifteen minutes
Yields: Twelve servings
Nutrition Facts: Calories: 123.3 | Protein: 2.9g | Carbs: 2.1g| Fat: 13.8g | Fiber: 1.1g

Ingredients

- Eight ounces of cream cheese (softened)
- One cup of cream
- One-third cup of sweetener
- One-fourth tsp. of stevia extract
- One tbsp. of lemon juice
- Two tsps. of lemon zest
- Two cups of strawberries (chopped)

Method:

1. Add the cream cheese in a food processor. Blend until smooth.

2. Add sweetener, cream, lemon zest, lemon juice, and stevia. Blend for one minute.

3. Add the strawberries. Process until smooth.

4. Pour the mixture into molds of popsicles.

5. Freeze for four hours.

Apple Cider Donut

Total Prep & Cooking Time: Thirty minutes
Yields: Twelve servings
Nutrition Facts: Calories: 162.3 | Protein: 7.2g |
Carbs: 3.9g| Fat: 14.7g | Fiber: 2.3g

Ingredients
For the donuts:
- Two cups of almond flour
- Half cup of sweetener
- One-fourth cup of each
    - Butter (melted)
    - Whey protein powder
- Two tsps. of baking powder
- Half tsp. of each
    - Salt
    - Cinnamon (ground)
- Two large eggs
- One-third cup of water
- Two tbsps. of each
    - Apple extract
    - Apple cider vinegar

For coating:
- One-fourth cup of sweetener
- Two tsps. of cinnamon (ground)
- Half cup of butter (melted)

Method:
1. Preheat your oven at one hundred and fifty
   degrees Celsius.

2. Use butter for greasing a mini muffin tray.

3. Combine all the listed ingredients for the donuts in a large bowl. Mix well.

4. Divide the donut mixture among the wells of the muffin tray.

5. Bake for twenty minutes. Remove the donuts. Let the donuts sit for five minutes.

6. Whisk the listed ingredients for the coating in a small bowl except for the melted butter.

7. Dip the donuts into the butter. Roll the donuts into the mixture of cinnamon.

8. Serve immediately.

Chapter 9: Easy Keto Dessert Recipes

No meal is regarded as complete without a tasty dessert. So, I have included some easy-to-make keto dessert recipes for you in this chapter.

Chocolate Cake

Total Prep & Cooking Time: One hour and thirty minutes
Yields: Twelve servings
Nutrition Facts: Calories: 322.3 | Protein: 7.6g | Carbs: 6.6g| Fat: 30.6g | Fiber: 4.9g

Ingredients
- Butter (for the pan)
- Four large eggs
- Half cup of each
  - Butter (unsalted)
  - Cocoa powder
- Two tsps. of stevia
- One tsp. of vanilla extract
- One cup of almond flour
- Half tsp. of each
  - Baking soda
  - Kosher salt

For the frosting:
- Half cup of butter (unsalted, softened)
- One-fourth cup of each

- o   Heavy cream
- o   Cocoa powder
- One tsp. of vanilla extract
- Two tsps. of stevia

Method:

1. Preheat your oven at one hundred and fifty degrees Celsius.

2. Use butter for greasing a baking dish.

3. Combine melted butter, eggs, vanilla extract, and stevia in a bowl.

4. Add cocoa powder and almond flour.

5. Add baking soda and salt. Mix well.

6. Transfer the batter of cake into the greased baking dish. Bake for twenty minutes.

7. Let the cake sit for one hour.

8. Whisk together all the listed ingredients for the frosting in a bowl.

9. Add the frosting on the cake. Spread properly.

10. Cut the cake in slices.

Keto Ice Cream

Total Prep & Cooking Time: Eight hours and fifteen minutes
Yields: Eight servings
Nutrition Facts: Calories: 340.3 | Protein: 2.6g | Carbs: 2.2g| Fat: 37.9g | Fiber: 0.3g

Ingredients
- Two cans of coconut milk
- Two cups of heavy cream
- One-fourth cup of confectioner's sweetener
- One tsp. of vanilla extract
- One pinch of kosher salt

Method:
1. Chill the coconut milk for three hours in the refrigerator.

2. Beat the creamy coconut milk using a hand mixer.

3. Combine sweetener, vanilla extract, and heavy cream in a bowl.

4. Add the coconut cream into the mixture of cream and vanilla.

5. Pour the prepared mixture into a medium-sized loaf pan.

6. Chill in the freezer for five hours.

Keto Mug Cake

Total Prep & Cooking Time: Fifteen minutes
Yields: One serving
Nutrition Facts: Calories: 465.6 | Protein: 14.6g |
Carbs: 7.6g| Fat: 45.5g | Fiber: 7.1g

Ingredients

- Two tbsps. of butter
- One-fourth cup of almond flour
- Two and a half tbsp. of cocoa powder
- One large egg (beaten)
- Three tbsps. of chocolate chips
- One and a half tbsp. of brown sugar (granulated)
- Half tsp. of baking powder
- One pinch of salt
- One-third cup of whipped cream (to serve)

Method:

1. Microwave the butter for thirty seconds.

2. Combine all the listed ingredients in a mug, except for the cream.

3. Bake for two minutes.

4. Garnish with cream on top.

Pumpkin Pie

Total Prep & Cooking Time: Three hours and thirty minutes
Yields: Sixteen servings
Nutrition Facts: Calories: 136.6 | Protein: 4.7g | Carbs: 9.9g| Fat: 4.9g | Fiber: 2.5g

Ingredients
For the crust:
- Two cups of almond flour
- Three tbsps. of coconut flour
- One-fourth tsp. of each
    - Kosher salt
    - Baking powder
- Four tbsps. of butter (melted)
- One egg (beaten)

For the filling:
- One can of pumpkin puree
- One cup of heavy cream
- Half cup of brown sugar
- Three large eggs
- One tsp. of cinnamon (ground)
- One-third tsp. of ginger (ground)
- One-fourth tsp. of each
    - Cloves (ground)
    - Nutmeg (ground)
    - Kosher salt
- Three-fourth tsp. of vanilla extract
- Whipped cream (to serve)

Method:

1. Preheat your oven at one hundred and fifty degrees Celsius.

2. Combine coconut flour, baking powder, salt, and almond flour in a bowl. Add egg and butter. Mix well.

3. Press the crust dough into a pie plate. Pork holes in the crust using a fork.

4. Bake the crust for ten minutes.

5. Combine all the listed ingredients for the pie filling in a large bowl.

6. Pour the filling into the crust.

7. Bake for fifty minutes.

8. Let the pie cool down for one hour.

9. Garnish with whipped cream.

Peanut Butter and Chocolate Cookies

Total Prep & Cooking Time: One hour and thirty minutes
Yields: Twenty servings
Nutrition Facts: Calories: 128.9 | Protein: 2.9g | Carbs: 9.6g| Fat: 6.6g | Fiber: 1.9g

Ingredients
- Two cups of peanut butter (unsweetened)
- One cup of coconut flour
- One-fourth cup of brown sugar
- One tsp. of vanilla extract
- One pinch of kosher salt
- Two cups of chocolate chips (melted)
- One tbsp. of coconut oil

Method:
1. Combine coconut flour, peanut butter, vanilla extract, sugar, and salt in a bowl.

2. Use parchment paper for lining a baking tray.

3. Use a mini cookie scoop for making rounds of cookies from the dough. Arrange the cookies on the baking tray. Slightly flatten them using your hands. Freeze for one hour.

4. Combine coconut oil along with chocolate chips in a bowl.

5. Dip the peanut butter cookies into the melted chocolate.

6. Place in the refrigerator for ten minutes.

7. Serve immediately.

Keto Frosty

Total Prep & Cooking Time: Forty-five minutes
Yields: Four servings
Nutrition Facts: Calories: 318.6 | Protein: 2.3g |
Carbs: 3.6g| Fat: 35.3g | Fiber: 1.1g

Ingredients
- Two cups of whipping cream
- Two tbsps. of cocoa powder
- Three tbsps. of powdered sugar sweetener
- One tsp. of vanilla extract
- One pinch of kosher salt

Method:
1. Combine cocoa powder, cream, salt, sweetener, and vanilla extract in a bowl. Mix well.

2. Pour the mixture into a Ziploc bag.

3. Place in the freezer for thirty minutes.

4. Cut off a tip of the Ziploc bag. Pipe the frosty into serving bowls.

Keto Brownie

Total Prep & Cooking Time: One hour and twenty-five minutes
Yields: Sixteen servings
Nutrition Facts: Calories: 265.3 | Protein: 7.1g | Carbs: 8.2g| Fat: 22.3g | Fiber: 5.6g

Ingredients
- Four large eggs
- Two ripe avocados
- Half cup of butter (melted)
- Six tbsps. of peanut butter
- Two tsps. of baking powder
- Two-third cup of granulated sugar
- One cup of cocoa powder
- Three tsps. of vanilla extract
- One tsp. of kosher salt

Method:
1. Preheat your oven at one hundred and fifty degrees Celsius.

2. Use parchment paper for lining a square baking pan.

3. Combine all the listed ingredients in a high power blender.

4. Transfer the mixture to the baking pan.

5. Bake for thirty minutes.

6. Let the brownie sit for thirty minutes.

7. Slice the brownie.

Keto Double Choco Muffin

Total Prep & Cooking Time: Twenty-five minutes
Yields: Six servings
Nutrition Facts: Calories: 278.3 | Protein: 7.2g |
Carbs: 6.7g| Fat: 28.3g | Fiber: 4.3g

Ingredients

- Two cups of almond flour
- Three-fourth cup of cocoa powder
- One-fourth cup of swerve sweetener
- Two tsps. of baking powder
- One tsp. of salt
- One cup of butter (melted)
- Three large eggs
- One and a half tsp. of vanilla extract
- One and a half cup of chocolate chips

Method:

1. Preheat your oven at one hundred and fifty degrees Celsius.

2. Use liners for lining a muffin pan.

3. Combine cocoa powder, sweetener, almond flour, baking powder, and salt.

4. Add eggs, vanilla extract, and butter. Mix well.

5. Add the chocolate mix.

6. Divide the prepared batter among the muffin cups.

7. Bake for twelve minutes.

8. Serve warm.

Avocado Keto Pops

Total Prep & Cooking Time: Six hours and ten minutes
Yields: Ten servings
Nutrition Facts: Calories: 122.2 | Protein: 1.6g | Carbs: 4.9g| Fat: 13.2g | Fiber: 3.3g

Ingredients

- Three ripe avocados
- Two limes (juiced)
- Three tbsps. of swerve sweetener
- Three-fourth cup of coconut milk
- One tbsp. of coconut oil
- One cup of chocolate chips

Method:

1. Add lime juice, avocados, coconut milk, and sweetener in a food processor. Keep blending until smooth.

2. Divide the avocado mixture among the popsicle molds.

3. Freeze for six hours.

4. Combine coconut oil and chocolate chips in a bowl. Microwave the mixture for melting.

5. Dip the frozen popsicles into the molten chocolate. Keep in the refrigerator for five minutes.

6. Serve immediately.

Choco Truffles

Total Prep & Cooking Time: Thirty minutes
Yields: Ten servings
Nutrition Facts: Calories: 21.3 | Protein: 2.3g | Carbs: 1.2g| Fat: 2.6g | Fiber: 0.9g

Ingredients
- One cup of dark chocolate chips (melted)
- One avocado (mashed)
- One tsp. of vanilla extract
- One-fourth tsp. of kosher salt
- One-fourth cup of cocoa powder

Method:
1. Combine avocado, melted chocolate, salt, and vanilla in a bowl. Mix well for making a smooth mixture.

2. Keep in the refrigerator for fifteen minutes.

3. Use a mini cookie scoop for scooping out one tbsp. of the mixture. Roll the mixture in small balls. Coat the balls in cocoa powder.

4. Serve immediately.

Carrot Cake Balls

Total Prep & Cooking Time: Fifteen minutes
Yields: Sixteen servings
Nutrition Facts: Calories: 125.6 | Protein: 2.3g |
Carbs: 5.4g| Fat: 12.6g | Fiber: 3.2g

Ingredients
- Eight ounces of cream cheese (softened)
- Three-fourth cup of coconut flour
- One tsp. of stevia
- Half tsp. of vanilla extract
- One and a half tsp. of cinnamon (ground)
- One-fourth tsp. of nutmeg (ground)
- Half cup of pecans (chopped)
- One cup of carrots (grated)
- One and a half cup of shredded coconut

Method:
1. Combine coconut flour, cream cheese, stevia, cinnamon, nutmeg, and vanilla in a bowl. Use a hand mixer for proper mixing.

2. Add the carrots. Fold the pecans.

3. Roll the mixture into small balls. Coat them in the shredded coconut.

4. Keep in the refrigerator for five minutes.

Blueberry Chocolate Clusters

Total Prep & Cooking Time: Twenty-five minutes
Yields: Fifteen servings
Nutrition Facts: Calories: 129.6 | Protein: 2.4g |
Carbs: 7.7g| Fat: 6.7g | Fiber: 1.3g

Ingredients
- Two cups of chocolate chips (melted)
- One tbsp. of coconut oil
- Two and a half cup of blueberries
- Flaky sea salt (to garnish)

Method:
1. Use parchment paper for lining a baking tray.

2. Melt the chocolate chips in a bowl with the coconut oil.

3. Add a dollop of the melted chocolate on the parchment paper.

4. Top the chocolate with five blueberries. Drizzle melted chocolate from the top. Sprinkle some sea salt.

5. Keep in the refrigerator for ten minutes.

6. Serve immediately.

Strawberry Cubes Covered With Chocolate

Total Prep & Cooking Time: Four hours and ten minutes
Yields: Eight servings
Nutrition Facts: Calories: 82.3 | Protein: 2.6g | Carbs: 7.1g| Fat: 7.6g | Fiber: 3.3g

Ingredients
- Two cups of chocolate chips
- Two tbsps. of coconut oil
- Sixteen strawberries (stems intact)

Method:
1. Melt chocolate chips along with coconut oil in a bowl.

2. Add a layer of melted chocolate at the base of an ice cube mold.

3. Top each cube with strawberry. Keep the stem side up.

4. Spoon remaining chocolate over the strawberries.

5. Keep in the refrigerator for four hours.

6. Serve immediately.

Tres Leches Cake

Total Prep & Cooking Time: Three hours and ten minutes
Yields: Eight servings
Nutrition Facts: Calories: 225.3 | Protein: 7.3g | Carbs: 2.1g| Fat: 22.1g | Fiber: 1.2g

Ingredients
For the cake:
- Three large eggs
- Four ounces of almond flour
- One tbsp. of coconut flour
- Two tbsps. of whipping cream
- One tsp. of baking powder
- Half tsp. of cream of tartar
- Three and a half ounce of erythritol
- Butter (for greasing)

For the sauce:
- Half cup of each
  - Whipping cream
  - Almond milk
- Three tbsps. of powdered erythritol
- One tbsp. of vanilla extract
- One pinch of salt
- Half tsp. of xanthan gum

For the cream:
- Half cup of whipping cream
- One tsp. of cream cheese
- Two tsps. of powdered erythritol

- One tsp. of cinnamon (ground, to serve)

Method:
1. Combine the listed ingredients for the cake.

2. Use butter for greasing a baking dish.

3. Pour the cake batter in the dish. Smoothen the top.

4. Microwave the cake for four minutes. Remove the cake from the microwave. Check if the cake is properly cooked in the center. If not, microwave again for three minutes. Repeat the process until the cake is properly cooked.

5. Combine all the ingredients for the sauce in a bowl. Mix well.

6. Combine the listed cream ingredients in a bowl using an electric mixer except for the cinnamon.

7. Use a fork for poking even holes on top of the cake. Add the sauce over the top surface. Refrigerate the cake for two hours.

8. Cover the cake surface with the cream.

9. Garnish with cinnamon.

Goat Cheese With Roasted Pistachios and Blackberries

Total Prep & Cooking Time: Thirty minutes
Yields: Four servings
Nutrition Facts: Calories: 582.3 | Protein: 34.3g |
Carbs: 4.2g| Fat: 47.1g | Fiber: 4.2g

Ingredients
- Twenty ounces of goat cheese

For the blackberry sauce:
- Nine ounces of blackberries
- One tbsp. of erythritol
- One pinch of cinnamon (ground)

For the topping:
- One ounce of pistachio nuts
- Salt
- Rosemary

Method:
1. Preheat your oven at one hundred and eighty degrees Celsius.

2. Mix cinnamon, blackberries, and sweetener.

3. Bake the goat cheese for twelve minutes.

4. Chop the pistachio nuts. Roast the nuts in a pan. Add some salt and toss.

5. Serve the goat cheese with roasted pistachios,
    blackberry, and rosemary.

Mocha Peppermint Ice Cream

Total Prep & Cooking Time: Three hours and fifteen minutes
Yields: Six servings
Nutrition Facts: Calories: 395.6 | Protein: 6.3g | Carbs: 4.2g| Fat: 36.3g | Fiber: 2.1g

Ingredients
- Two cups of whipping cream
- Two ounces of dark chocolate (chopped)
- Six large egg yolks
- Two-third cup of powdered erythritol
- Two tbsps. of coffee powder
- Two tsps. of vanilla extract
- Half tsp. of salt
- One pinch of peppermint extract
- Six drops of sweetener

Method:
1. Heat the whipping cream in a large pan.

2. Add the chopped chocolate. Keep stirring until the chocolate melts.

3. Add the egg yolks in the pan.

4. Add powdered sweetener along with the coffee powder. Keep whisking for ten minutes on low heat until the mixture thickens. Make sure the yolks do not get cooked.

5. Remove the pan from the heat. Add salt, peppermint, and vanilla extract.

6. Pour the mixture in an air-tight container. Freeze for three hours.

7. Scoop out the frozen ice cream in serving bowls.

8. Serve immediately.

Spicy Gingerbread Dutch Baby

Total Prep & Cooking Time: Thirty minutes
Yields: Six servings
Nutrition Facts: Calories: 247.3 | Protein: 8.1g |
Carbs: 2.2g| Fat: 22.3g | Fiber: 0.3g

Ingredients
- Three-fourth cup of whipping cream
- Five large eggs
- Two ounces of cream cheese (softened)
- One tsp. of vanilla extract
- Half tsp. of maple extract
- One-third cup of powdered erythritol
- Two tbsps. of whey protein powder
- Two tsps. of baking powder
- One-fourth tsp. of salt
- One-third tsp. of ginger (ground)
- Three-fourth tsp. of each
    - Cloves (ground)
    - Cinnamon (ground)
- Three tbsps. of butter

Method:
1. Preheat your oven at two hundred degrees Celsius.

2. Add all the listed ingredients in a food processor except for the butter. Blend the ingredients for two minutes.

3. Add the butter in a skillet. Place the skillet in the oven.

4. Remove the pan from the oven as the butter starts sizzling.

5. Add the batter in the skillet.

6. Bake for fifteen minutes.

No-Bake Chocolate Cake

Total Prep & Cooking Time: One hour and twenty minutes
Yields: Twelve servings
Nutrition Facts: Calories: 401.3 | Protein: 8.3g |
Carbs: 4.1g| Fat: 38.9g | Fiber: 5.2g

Ingredients
- Two cups of whipping cream
- Three tbsps. of erythritol
- Seven ounces of dark chocolate
- Four ounces of butter
- One pinch of salt
- Seven ounces of hazelnuts
- Three and a half ounce of pumpkin seeds

Method:
1. Boil cream and sweetener in a pan. Let the mixture simmer for two minutes.

2. Chop the butter along with the chocolate into smaller pieces. Add them to the pan. Stir for melting. Add salt.

3. Roast the pumpkin seeds along with hazelnuts in a pan.

4. Chop the nut mixture. Add it to the pan.

5. Add the mixture of chocolate into a springform pan. Cover the pan.

6. Refrigerate for one hour.

Keto Cheesecake

Total Prep & Cooking Time: One hour and thirty minutes
Yields: Twelve servings
Nutrition Facts: Calories: 345.2 | Protein: 6.8g | Carbs: 4.1g| Fat: 34.3g | Fiber: 0.2g

Ingredients
For the crust:
- Two cups of almond flour
- Two ounces of butter
- Two tbsps. of erythritol
- Half tsp. of vanilla extract

For the filling:
- Twenty ounces of cream cheese
- Half cup of whipping cream
- Two large eggs
- One egg yolk
- One tbsp. of erythritol
- One tsp. of lemon zest
- Half tsp. of vanilla extract
- Two ounces of blueberries

Method:
1. Preheat your oven at one hundred and eighty degrees Celsius.

2. Use parchment paper for lining the springform pan base.

3. Heat butter for the crust in a pan.

4. Remove the pan from heat. Add sweetener, vanilla, and almond flour.

5. Press the dough into the pan base.

6. Bake for eight minutes.

7. Combine all the listed ingredients for the filling in a large bowl.

8. Pour the mixture for the filling into the crust.

9. Bake the cake for fifteen minutes at a temperature of two hundred degrees Celsius.

10. Reduce the temperature to one hundred degrees Celsius. Bake for one hour.

11. Serve with blueberries on top.

Rhubarb Tart

Total Prep & Cooking Time: One hour and five minutes
Yields: Eight servings
Nutrition Facts: Calories: 510.3 | Protein: 10.6g | Carbs: 3.3g| Fat: 50.3g | Fiber: 1.3g

Ingredients
For the crust:
- Six ounces of almond flour
- One-third cup of erythritol
- One ounce of shredded coconut
- Three ounces of butter

For the almond cream filling:
- Five ounces of butter (softened)
- Half cup of erythritol
- Two cups of almond flour
- Three large eggs
- One tsp. of vanilla extract
- Seven ounces of rhubarb

Method:
1. Preheat your oven at one hundred and eighty degrees Celsius.

2. Grease a tart pan with butter.

3. Melt the butter in a saucepan.

4. Combine all the listed dry ingredients with the melted butter.

5. Add the crust dough in the pan. Press the prepared dough along the base and the sides of the pan.

6. Bake for ten minutes.

7. Combine erythritol and butter in a bowl. Add eggs, almond flour, and vanilla extract. Mix well.

8. Peel thin and long strips from the stalks of rhubarb.

9. Add the filling into the crust.

10. Make spirals from the strips of rhubarb. Push the spirals into the tart filling.

11. Bake the tart for thirty minutes.

Keto Waffles and Blueberry Butter

Total Prep & Cooking Time: Fifteen minutes
Yields: Four servings
Nutrition Facts: Calories: 570.3 | Protein: 15.2g |
Carbs: 3.1g| Fat: 55.6g | Fiber: 4.6g

Ingredients

- Five ounces of butter (melted)
- Eight large eggs
- One tsp. of vanilla extract
- Two tsps. of baking powder
- One-third cup of coconut flour

For the blueberry butter:

- Three ounces of butter
- One ounce of blueberries

Method:

1. Combine eggs along with melted butter in a bowl. Add the remaining listed ingredients. Use a hand mixer for smooth mixing.

2. Heat a waffle iron.

3. Add the waffle batter into the waffle iron. Cook for four minutes. Repeat with the remaining batter.

4. Combine blueberries and butter in a bowl. Use an electric mixer for proper mixing.

5. Serve the waffles with blueberry butter on top.

Vanilla Ice Cream

Total Prep & Cooking Time: Two hours and twenty minutes
Yields: Six servings
Nutrition Facts: Calories: 256.6 | Protein: 7.9g | Carbs: 2.9g| Fat: 26.3g | Fiber: 0.3g

Ingredients

- Six egg yolks
- One cup of coconut milk
- Two cups of almond milk
- One-third cup of xylitol
- Half cup of avocado oil
- Two tsps. of vanilla extract
- One-eighth tsp. of salt

Method:

1. Heat almond milk along with coconut milk in a pan. Add the egg yolks. Keep stirring until the mixture thickens.

2. Add the sweetener. Whisk for ten minutes.

3. Remove the pan from heat.

4. Add vanilla extract, oil, and salt. Add the mixture in a blender. Blend for thirty seconds.

5. Pour the mixture in an air-tight container.

6. Freeze the ice cream for two hours.

Lemon Ice Cream

Total Prep & Cooking Time: Two hours and thirty minutes
Yields: Six servings
Nutrition Facts: Calories: 270.3 | Protein: 5.1g | Carbs: 3.2g| Fat: 26.6g | Fiber: 0.6g

Ingredients

- One lemon (juiced, zested)
- Three large eggs
- One-third cup of erythritol
- Two cups of whipping cream
- One-fourth tsp. of yellow food coloring

Method:

1. Separate the egg whites from the yolks.

2. Beat the whites until stiff.

3. Combine sweetener and egg yolks in a bowl. Add the lemon juice. Add the food coloring. Mix well.

4. Add the egg whites gently into the lemon and egg yolk mixture.

5. Whip the cream until it forms soft peaks.

6. Fold the mixture of eggs into the whipped cream.

7. Pour the mixture of ice cream into an air-tight container.

8. Freeze for two hours.

**Vanilla Panna Cotta**

Total Prep & Cooking Time: Three hours and ten minutes
Yields: Four servings
Nutrition Facts: Calories: 423.6 | Protein: 4.6g | Carbs: 3.8g| Fat: 44.3g | Fiber: 0.2g

Ingredients

- Two tsps. of powdered gelatin
- Water
- Two cups of whipping cream
- One tbsp. of vanilla extract
- One tsp. of erythritol
- Two tbsps. of pomegranates

Method:

1. Mix gelatin in cold water according to the packet instructions.

2. Combine vanilla extract, cream, and erythritol in a pan. Boil the mixture.

3. Simmer the mixture for five minutes.

4. Remove the pan from the heat. Add the gelatin. Mix well.

5. Divide the cream mixture into serving glasses.

6. Cover the glasses with cling wrap.

7. Keep in the refrigerator for three hours.

8. Serve with pomegranates on top.

Mason Jar Ice Cream

Total Prep & Cooking Time: One hour and ten minutes
Yields: One serving
Nutrition Facts: Calories: 470.3 | Protein: 6.3g | Carbs: 4.6g| Fat: 48.7g | Fiber: 0.3g

Ingredients
- Half cup of whipping cream
- One egg yolk
- One tbsp. of erythritol
- Half tsp. of vanilla extract

Method:
1. Add all the listed ingredients in a mason jar. Close the lid.

2. Shake the jar vigorously for five minutes.

3. Chill in the freezer for one hour.

Conclusion

I want to thank you for reaching the end of *Keto Diet After 50*. I hope it was full of useful information and capable of providing you all the tools you will require to achieve all the goals.

Now, all you have to do is start with the keto meal plan from the coming week. The quicker you start with the diet plan, the faster you can see the results. Do not just sit and try to figure out the perfect day for starting with the diet. This way, you can never start with the diet plan. If you are waiting for the perfect day, then it is today. As soon as you start with twenty-one days keto meal plan, try your best not to deflect. It is not that tough. Cutting out carbs suddenly might seem to be a bit tough at the beginning. However, once you see the diet plan results after three weeks, you will be amazed. There is nothing too complex about the ketogenic diet. Life after the age of 50 is not at all easy. It will be better for you if you start aiding all the problems from the very beginning.

Just take your grocery bag and go out shopping for all the items that you will need. You can create a shopping list according to the diet meal plan for each week. It will make your task a lot easier. The keto diet has shown positive results after the age of fifties. The recipes that I have included in this book, apart from the keto meal plan recipes, are very easy. You can gather the ingredients from your local grocery store.

So, what are you waiting for? Start preparing healthy meals and lead a healthy life after your fifties.

Finally, if this book could help you in any way, kindly leave an Amazon review.